An Aid to the MRCP:
Essential Lists, Facts and Mnemonics

This book is due for return on or before the last date shown below.

19 JAN 2012

13 JAN 2009   17 MAY 2011

17 JUL 2009

      15 JUN 2011

4 - MAY 2010   2 5 JUL 2011

18 - JuL 2011

3 AUG 2010   17.02.17

- 7 SEP 2010

04.01.2011

17/1/11

7 DAY LOAN

An Aid to the MRCP
Essential Lists, Facts and Mnemonics

Nicholas K. Boeckx
West Midlands

R. E. J. Ryder
Department of Medicine
City Hospital
Birmingham

M. A. Mir
Department of Integrated Medicine
Royal Gwent and St Woolos Hospitals
Newport Gwent

E. A. Freeman
Department of Medicine
University of Wales College of Medicine
Cardiff

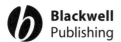

Blackwell
Publishing

© 2008 Nicholas K. Boeckx, R. E. J. Ryder, M. A. Mir, E. A. Freeman
Published by Blackwell Publishing
Blackwell Publishing, Inc., 350 Main Street, Malden, Massachusetts 02148–5020, USA
Blackwell Publishing Ltd, 9600 Garsington Road, Oxford OX4 2DQ, UK
Blackwell Publishing Asia Pty Ltd, 550 Swanston Street, Carlton, Victoria 3053, Australia

First published 2008

1 2008

Library of Congress Cataloging-in-Publication Data

An aid to the MRCP : essential lists, facts and mnemonics / Nicholas K. Boeckx . . . [et al.].
    p. ; cm.
  Includes index.
  ISBN 978-1-4051-7650-7
  1. Internal medicine–Examinations, questions, etc.   2. Diagnosis–Examinations, questions, etc.
3. Physicians–Licenses–Great Britain–Examinations–Study guides.   I. Boeckx, Nicholas K.
  [DNLM: 1. Diagnosis, Differential–Programmed Instruction.   2. Physical Examination–
Programmed Instruction.   WB 18.2 A2875 2008]

  RC58.A35 2008
  616.0076–dc22   2007021628

A catalogue record for this title is available from the British Library

Set in 8/11 pt Frutiger by SNP Best-set Typesetter Ltd., Hong Kong
Printed and bound in Singapore by Utopia Press Pte Ltd

Commissioning Editor: Alison Brown
Editorial Assistant: Jennifer Seward
Development Editor: Fiona Pattison
Production Controller: Debbie Wyer

For further information on Blackwell Publishing, visit our website:
http://www.blackwellpublishing.com

The publisher's policy is to use permanent paper from mills that operate a sustainable forestry policy,
and which has been manufactured from pulp processed using acid-free and elementary chlorine-free
practices. Furthermore, the publisher ensures that the text paper and cover board used have met
acceptable environmental accreditation standards.

Contents

Introduction

The MRCP exam is a difficult challenge and this book aims to give you the best chance of passing (first time). In order to pass you will need to learn a large number of lists and key facts. This book provides the essential lists and facts that you need to know together with memory aids to speed learning and recall. Armed with this knowledge you will be able to rapidly narrow your differential diagnosis and identify the most likely answer. Using this technique NKB passed all parts of the MRCP on his first attempt.

The lists in this book and the mnemonics that accompany them include only information likely to present in the exam. Where possible the memory aids are related to the topic.

Each of the memory aids, facts and lists in this book is based on questions faced while revising for, or encountered during, the MRCP exams.

Acknowledgements

Thank you to everyone involved with this revision text. In particular I would like to thank my wife, my friends and my colleagues who have spent their time reading and reviewing for me. Special thanks go to Jill Boeckx, Jo Kirby, Alison Brown and my family.

Nicholas K. Boeckx

Page layout

The topic category is listed at the side of the page and topic at the page head. Below the topic heading is a memory aid and explanation. Topic facts are listed beneath this heading.

Topic   Mnemonic   Category

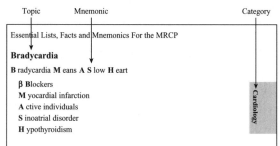

Essential Lists, Facts and Mnemonics For the MRCP

Bradycardia

B radycardia **M** eans **A** **S** low **H** eart

β **B**lockers
M yocardial infarction
A ctive individuals
S inoatrial disorder
H ypothyroidism

Cardiology

Topic facts
Sinus bradycardia is defined as a heart rate <60 beats/min. The common causes are listed above.

• β Blockade is the most common cause of sinus bradycardia seen in hospital patients.

• Very fit individuals may have a slow resting heart rate.

• Heart block is suggested by a heart rate<40 beats/min. An ECG trace will show a dissociation between the 'p' waves and the QRS complexes. QRS complexes are broad because the focus is in the ventricles. Cannon waves (atrial contraction against a closed tricuspid valve) may be seen in complete heart block as a result of loss of synchronicity between atria and ventricles.

• Heart rate is the best clinical indicator of thyroid status (i.e.under-/over-active). Other indicators of thyroid status are:

   – tremor
   – sweaty palms
   – reflexes (test ankle)
   – AF
   – thyroid bruit
   – lid lag.

Candidates should be aware that most thyroid patients presented will be euthyroid. The presence of eye signs does not indicate hyperthyroidism–patients with Graves' disease may be hyper-, hypo- or euthyroid.

Errors and additions

Every effort has been made to ensure accuracy; however, if you spot any mistakes or have any suggestions for the next edition please contact NKB at anaidtothemrcp@hotmail.co.uk.

Audio revision

To make the best use of your time, why not download the free audio revision tool at www.anaidtothemrcp.com. Use the time you spend commuting to improve your knowledge for the exam. The revision tool is based on a summary of the mnemonics contained in this book.

Haematology

- Anaemia (categorized by cell size)
- Anaemia – congenital haemolytic
- Anticoagulants
- Bleeding disorders
- Eosinophilia
- High erythrocyte sedimentation rate (ESR)
- Immunodeficiency
- Leukaemia – acute lymphoblastic leukaemia (ALL)
- Leukaemia – chronic lymphatic leukaemia (CLL)
- Leukaemia – chronic myeloid leukaemia (CML)
- Microangiopathic haemolytic anaemia (MHA)
- Pancytopenia
- Polycythaemia
- Thrombocytosis
- Thrombosis
- Warfarin and heparin

Anaemia – categorized by cell size

Microcytic
Small **T**ypically **I**ron
  Sideroblastic
  Thalassaemia
  Iron deficiency

Macrocytic
My **B**lood **H**as **L**arge **E**rythrocytes
  Myelodysplasia
  B$_{12}$ deficiency
  Haemolysis
  Liver disease
  Embryo (pregnancy)

Normocytic
Exclude **C**hronic **A**naemia
  Endocrine (hypopituitary, thyroid, adrenal)
  Combined deficiency
  Acute blood loss/**A**plastic

Topic facts
This mnemonic lists the causes of anaemia categorized by cell size into microcytic, macrocytic and normocytic. These correspond to mean corpuscular or cell volume (MCV) of <76, 76–96 and >96 fL, respectively.
- Hypothyroidism commonly causes macrocytosis but can also cause a normocytic anaemia.
- An MCV >110 fL is most likely to be caused by vitamin B$_{12}$ or folate deficiency.
- Thalassaemia trait presents with microcytosis and a high red cell count (typically >5 × 10^9/L).
- Chronic disease that typically causes a normocytic anaemia (e.g. cancer, rheumatic disease).

Anaemia – congenital haemolytic
Membrane/Enzyme/Haemoglobin

Membrane
Spherocytosis
Elliptocytosis

Enzyme
Glucose-6-phosphate dehydrogenase (G6PD) deficiency

Haemoglobin
Thalassaemia
Sickle cell disease

Topic facts
This topic divides the causes of congenital haemolytic anaemia into three categories: defects of the cell membrane, the cell enzymes and haemoglobin.

- Congenital haemolytic anaemia is suggested by a positive family history and the triad of anaemia, splenomegaly and jaundice.
- Hereditary spherocytosis is the most common of the congenital haemolytic anaemias. It has autosomal dominant inheritance.
- Precipitants of a haemolytic episode include infection and oxidative stress (especially drugs such as dapsone, quinine and nitrofurantoin).
- Investigation of haemolytic anaemia: blood film (for spherocytes, elliptocytes), direct Coombs' test (for autoimmune haemolysis), G6PD assay.
- Patients with severe anaemia may require splenectomy.
- G6PD deficiency leads to haemolysis of red blood cells when they are exposed to oxidative stress. In normal cells G6PD maintains levels of the important antioxidant glutathione.

Anticoagulants

APTT

   Anti-thrombin 3
   Proteins C + S

Topic facts

APTT stands for **a**ctivated **p**artial **t**hromboplastin **t**ime – a measure of clotting time. This abbreviation can be used to help recall the body's natural anticoagulants anti-thrombin 3 and proteins C + S.

- The body contains a natural anticoagulant mechanism made up of three factors: anti-thrombin 3, protein C and protein S. Thrombophilic states arise as a result of a deficiency or impaired function of one or more of these factors.

- Factor V Leiden mutation is the most common thrombophilic state. It is caused by a genetic abnormality of clotting factor 5. As a result of the mutation, protein C cannot bind to factor 5 and inactivate the clotting cascade. It has autosomal dominant inheritance.

- Factor V Leiden is investigated by using a PCR (polymerase chain reaction) to identify the abnormal gene or by the activated protein C resistance test. (Protein C is added to a sample of patient's plasma and the APTT is measured. In a normal individual, addition of the natural anticoagulant protein C prolongs the clotting time. In individuals with factor V Leiden protein C is unable to bind and the APTT is unchanged.)

- Isolated protein C and protein S deficiencies are less common. They are both inherited as autosomal dominant conditions. Most patients are identified on thrombophilia screening after recurrent deep vein thrombosis.

- Anti-thrombin 3 deficiency may result as a complication of nephrotic syndrome. Patients with nephrotic syndrome are at risk of arterial and venous thrombosis due to a loss of anti-thrombin 3 in the kidneys.

Bleeding disorders
Capillary/Platelet/Coagulation

Capillary
Inherited
- Collagen diseases (page 161)
- Hereditary haemorrhagic telangiectasia

Acquired
- Severe infection
- Purpuras (senile, steroid, Henoch–Schönlein)

Platelet
- ITP (idiopathic thrombocytopenic purpura – young females ± splenomegaly)
- Marrow infiltration (secondaries, leukaemia)
- Marrow aplasia (drugs, viral)

Coagulation
- Anticoagulant treatment
- Haemophilia A or B
- Von Willebrand's disease

Topic facts
This topic covers disorders that cause excessive bleeding. They are best divided into capillary, platelet and coagulation defects. A clinical hallmark of excessive bleeding is bruising (purpura).
- Von Willebrand's disease is the most common bleeding disorder in the UK. It is an autosomal dominant condition, resulting from an abnormality of chromosome 12.
- Von Willebrand's factor is important for the adhesion of platelets to damaged blood vessel walls. Patients present with excessive bruising, menorrhagia and epistaxis.
- Patients with haemophilia A (X-linked recessive inheritance) lack factor 8. Patients with haemophilia B (Christmas disease) lack factor 9.

Eosinophilia

Severe eosinophilia >5 × 10⁹/L

Painful **B**listers
   Parasitic infection
   Blistering skin diseases

Severe eosinophilia >5 × 10⁹/L + abnormal chest radiograph

High **E**osinophils + **L**ung **T**rouble
   Hypereosinophilic syndrome
   Eosinophilic pneumonia
   Leukaemia (eosinophilic)
   Tropical pulmonary eosinophilia

Topic facts

Severe eosinophilia is defined as >5 × 10^9/L eosinophils. The causes of a severe eosinophilia can be divided into patients with and those without lung involvement.

- Other causes of eosinophilia to be considered include allergies, Churg–Strauss vasculitis and Hodgkin's lymphoma. These typically cause a less severe eosinophilia (0.5–2.0 × 10^9/L).
- The blistering skin diseases are pemphigoid, pemphigus and erythema multiforme (nb dermatitis herpenfarmis is a blistering skin disease which causes a less severe eosinophilia).
- Parasites associated with eosinophilia include *Strongyloides*, *Filariasis* and *Ascaris* and *Wuchereria bancrofti*. Parasitic eosinophilia is not common in the UK.
- Hypereosinophilic syndrome patients have the triad of eosinophilia, restrictive cardiomyopathy and hepatosplenomegaly.
- Allergies causing eosinophilia include both allergic conditions, such as asthma and allergic rhinitis, and drug allergies (particularly sulfonamides and nitrofurantoin).

High erythrocyte sedimentation rate (ESR) (>100 mm/h)

Vasculitis **M**ay **P**rolong **S**edimentation

Vasculitis
Myeloma
Polymyalgia rheumatica
Sepsis

Topic facts

This topic lists the causes of a very high ESR defined as >100 mm/h.

- ESR is a measure of the rate at which red blood cells settle in a blood specimen.
- The rate of sedimentation is affected by several factors, the most important of which is the concentration of proteins in the blood. Protein levels rise in the blood during inflammation as a result of the acute phase response. Fibrinogen, a major acute phase reactant, is an important cause of the increase in sedimentation rate during inflammation.
- Proteins other than acute phase reactants cause elevation of the ESR. High plasma concentrations of immunoglobulins, caused by myeloma or paraproteinaemias, are examples of this.
- The ESR is also affected by the size and shape of the red blood cells. Thus anaemia, old age and pregnancy can lead to an elevation in ESR.
- Polymyalgia rheumatica is characterized by an ESR >100 mm/h and pain and stiffness of the shoulder and pelvic girdles. It is rare before the age of 50 and is associated with giant cell arteritis. Muscle weakness is NOT a feature of polymyalgia; if this is present suspect polymyositis. Treatment is with high-dose steroids.
- Myeloma is a disease of elderly people. The high levels of immunoglobulins cause hyperviscosity and elevation of the ESR. Patients are at risk of arterial and venous thrombosis.

Immunodeficiency

Drugs **M**ay **C**ause **L**owered **I**mmunity

Drugs

Myeloma

Common variable hypogammaglobulinaemia

Lymphoma/**L**eukaemia (CLL)

Infection (HIV)

Topic facts

This mnemonic provides a simplified list of the more common causes of immunodeficiency, which can be categorized into primary (common variable) and secondary (the rest). There are many rare esoteric eponymous primary disorders, but time spent learning these may be better used revising other topics.

- Drug-induced hypogammaglobulinaemia is caused by agents such as phenytoin and penicillamine.
- Myeloma patients have high levels of monoclonal γ-globulins. These have an immunoparetic effect by suppressing the body's immune response to antigens.
- The immunosuppressive effect of immunoglobulins can be used therapeutically in patients with autoimmune disorders. Intravenous immunoglobulin is used to suppress the harmful autoimmune response, e.g. in Guillain–Barré syndrome.
- Common variable hypogammaglobulinaemia is a primary immunodeficiency disorder. Patients have low levels of antibody and a history of recurrent bacterial and fungal infections.
- Haematological neoplasms such as lymphoma and chronic lymphocytic leukaemia are associated with hypogammaglobulinaemia.
- HIV infection leads to impaired cell-mediated immunity through its effect on CD4 T-helper cells.
- Hypogammaglobulinaemia can complicate nephrotic syndrome through renal loss of antibodies.

Leukaemia – Acute lymphoblastic leukaemia (ALL)

ALL the kids respond (to treatment).

Topic facts

Acute lymphoblastic leukaemia (ALL) is the most common malignancy in children. More than 90 per cent will respond to treatment (with cure rates of around 70 per cent).

- Leukaemias (the bone marrow malignancies) are classified by the cell type and degree of maturity of the cells.
- Acute leukaemias are associated with immature blast cells and rapid disease progression.
- Chronic leukaemias have more mature leukocytes and a slow rate of disease progression.
- Suspect chronic leukaemia in patients with a high white cell count (WCC) (typical values: chronic myeloid leukaemia (CML) >50 neutrophils, chronic lympharic lymphocytic leukaemia (CLL) >15 lymphocytes).
- In acute leukaemia the WCC may be raised, normal or low. The blast cells seen on the blood film, which are very large (approximately four times the size of red blood cells), are the key feature.
- Acute myeloid leukaemia (AML) can be differentiated from ALL under the microscope by the presence of Auer rods (which are small inclusion bodies).
- Patients with acute leukaemia present with the features of bone marrow failure, i.e. infection, anaemia and bleeding.

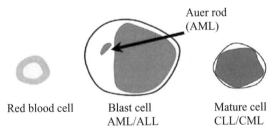

Auer rod
(AML)

Red blood cell   Blast cell   Mature cell
                 AML/ALL   CLL/CML

Chronic Myeloid Leukaemia

A diagram showing the relative sizes and appearances of blood cells on a blood film.

Leukaemia – Chronic lymphatic leukaemia (CLL)

B disease
    B lymphocytes (95 per cent)
    Bone marrow failure
    Bleeding
    Broken cells (smear cells)

Topic facts

This mnemonic summarizes the pathology, presentation and blood film findings of chronic lymphatic leukaemia (CLL).

- CLL is the most common form of leukaemia affecting adults in the UK.
- Ninety-five per cent of CLL is of B-cell origin.
- CLL is most commonly found in the late middle-aged to elderly population.
- The disease proceeds through a number of stages. Initially patients are asymptomatic and the only feature may be lymphocytosis (high WCC). Subsequently lymphadenopathy develops, followed by hepatosplenomegaly and eventually bone marrow failure.
- Presenting symptoms are a result of bone marrow failure (anaemia, infection, bleeding).
- Patients may also complain of lethargy, weight loss and night sweats.
- Investigation is with a blood film and bone marrow.
- The blood film shows large numbers of mature lymphocytes.
- Increased fragility of the mature B-cell membranes causes a number of the cells to break open on preparation of a slide. These are called smear cells and are typical of CLL.
- First-line treatment is with chlorambucil.
- Patients with CLL are susceptible to folate deficiency caused by increased consumption as the result of rapid cell turnover.

Leukaemia – chronic myeloid leukaemia (CML)

Myeloid **L**eukaemia **P**atient
   Middle age
   Leukoerythroblastic blood picture
   Philadelphia chromosome

Topic facts

The age of onset, blood film findings and pathology of chronic myeloid leukaemia (CML) are summarized in this mnemonic.

- CML is a myeloproliferative disorder in which there is increased turnover of the granulocyte cell line (neutrophils, basophils, eosinophils).
- The blood film shows high numbers of granulocytes and myeloid precursor cells (metamyelocytes, myelocytes). Nucleated red blood cells are also seen.
- The combination of myeloid precursors and nucleated red blood cells is termed a 'leukoerythroblastic picture' (also called a leukaemoid reaction).
- The causes of a leukoerythroblastic picture include bone marrow infiltration (leukaemia, lymphoma, myelofibrosis, other neoplasms) and severe stressors (sepsis, severe inflammation, tissue necrosis, haemorrhage).
- Almost all patients with CML are Philadelphia chromosome positive. The Philadelphia chromosome is created from a translocation of the long arms of chromosome 9 and 22 – t(9:22).
- You may be asked to differentiate between the diagnosis of CML and myelofibrosis in a patient presenting with splenomegaly and myeloid precursors. Both disorders present with a leukocytosis and leukoerythroblastic picture:
  - CML patients are Philadelphia chromosome positive (myelofibrosis patients are negative)
  - myelofibrosis patients have a high NAP (neutrophil alkaline phosphatase) score (CML patients have a low NAP score).

Microangiopathic haemolytic anaemia

Microangiopathic **H**aemolytic **A**naemia **C**auses **B**lood **V**essel **D**amage

Mucinous adenocarcinoma

HUS/TTP (haemolytic uraemic syndrome/thrombotic thrombocytopenic purpura)

Accelerated hypertension

Connective tissue diseases

Burns

Vasculitis

Disseminated intravascular coagulation (DIC)

A fibrin strand haemolysing a red blood cell into fragment (helmet) cells.

Topic facts

This topic covers the causes of microangiopathic haemolytic anaemia (MHA).

- MHA, as the name suggests, affects the small blood vessels. It damages the endothelial cell walls and causes fibrin strand deposition.
- The most common causes of MHA are DIC and HUS/TTP.
- The deposited fibrin strands slice open red blood cells as they pass through the vessel, resulting in a haemolytic anaemia. Some of the damaged red cells are able to reseal and are described on the blood film as fragment or helmet cells.
- Other haematological features include a high reticulocyte count and polychromasia.
- Suspect DIC in patients with prolonged coagulation times and high fibrinogen degradation products with a MHA blood picture. DIC prolongs all clotting times (APTT, INR [international normalized ratio], TT [thrombin time], BT [bleeding time]).
- HUS is associated with infection with *Escherichia coli*. A history of gastrointestinal symptoms, fever and renal impairment is highly suggestive.

Pancytopenia

Pancytopenia

My **S**pleen **I**njures **C**ells

Marrow infiltration

Spleen (hypersplenism)

Idiopathic acquired

Congenital (Fanconi's anaemia)

Pancytopenia with a raised MCV (>96 fL)

Impaired **M**arrow **P**roduces **S**ome **B**ig **C**ells

Infections (Epstein–Barr virus – [EBV])

Myxoedema/**M**yelodysplasia

Paroxysmal nocturnal haemoglobinuria (PNH)

Systemic lupus erythematosus (SLE)

B$_{12}$ and folate deficiency

Cytotoxics

Topic facts

There are two memory aids in this topic; they cover the more common causes of pancytopenia categorized by the presence or absence of a raised MCV, defined as >96 fL.

- Pancytopenia is defined as a deficiency of all of the blood cells (white cells, platelets and red cells). There are a large number of causes of pancytopenia and the most useful way to categorize them is by red cell size.
- Marrow infiltration includes lymphoma, leukaemia, myeloma and secondary metastasis to the bones.
- Fanconi's anaemia is a congenital autosomal recessive condition associated with bone marrow failure, developmental abnormalities and a reduced life expectancy.

✓ Polycythaemia
Primary/Secondary/Inappropriate

Primary
Polycythaemia rubra vera

Secondary (hypoxia driven)
Chronic lung disease
Right-to-left cardiac shunts (often congenital)
High altitude

Inappropriate
Tumours: renal, liver, brain

Topic facts
Polycythaemia is defined as an elevated haemoglobin, red cell count and packed cell volume (PCV). The causes of polycythaemia are best categorized into primary, secondary and inappropriate.

- Red cell production is regulated by the hormone erythropoietin, which is made in the kidney in response to tissue hypoxia.
- Primary polycythaemia is termed 'polycythaemia rubra vera' (PRV). There is uncontrolled production of red cells independent of erythropoietin. PRV is a myeloproliferative disorder.
- PRV patients typically have raised platelet and neutrophil counts (red cells, platelets and neutrophils come from the same myeloid line which is over-actively proliferating). Use this to help differentiate primary polycythaemia from other causes.
- Secondary causes of polycythaemia are a response to tissue hypoxia and elevated levels of erythropoietin. This can be thought of as appropriate polycythaemia.
- Inappropriate polycythaemia therefore refers to polycythaemia in which there are elevated erythropoietin levels in the absence of a hypoxic drive, e.g. erythropoietin-producing tumours.

Thrombocytosis

Massive **B**leeding **I**ncreases **P**latelet **C**ount **S**ignificantly

  Myeloproliferative disease

  Bleeding

  Inflammation/**I**ron deficiency

  Primary thrombocytosis

  Connective tissue disease/**C**ancer

  Splenectomy

Topic facts

Thrombocytosis (elevated platelet count) is defined as $>400 \times 10^9$/L. The causes are summarized as follows.

- Primary thrombocytosis (essential thrombocythaemia) patients typically have platelet counts above 1000×10^9/L. Associated features of myeloproliferative disease (polycythaemia, splenomegaly) help to differentiate it from secondary causes.
- Myeloproliferative disease is included as a separate heading because platelet counts can also rise in association with other myeloproliferative disorders such as PRV.
- The spleen is important in the destruction of platelets and thus levels may remain elevated post-splenectomy. The clue will be the presence of Howell–Jolly bodies in the blood film report.
- Thrombocytosis is commonly found in patients with iron deficiency. MRCP questions may provide a clue to this by reporting the blood film. Look for microcytosis, anisocytosis, poikilocytosis and hypochromasia. A picture of koilonychia (spooning of the nails) may be shown (however, this can be inherited as an autosomal dominant familial trait).
- Inflammation and bleeding cause a transient thrombocytosis.

Thrombosis

Pathologically **S**ticky **B**lood **T**hromboses **A**ll **V**essels

    Paroxysmal nocturnal haemoglobinuria (PNH)

    Sickle cell

    Behçet's syndrome

    Thrombophilia

    Antiphospholipid syndrome

    Vasculitides

Topic facts

The conditions that can cause both arterial and venous thrombosis are summarized in this topic.

- PNH is a rare, acquired disorder of red blood cells. The cell membranes are susceptible to lysis by the complement system. Patients present with dark urine and thrombosis. Haemolytic anaemia is present (low haemoglobin with a raised reticulocyte count). Ham's test is positive (red cell lysis in acidified serum).
- Sickle cell disease (HbSS) is an autosomal recessive disorder. HbSS causes sickling during deoxygenation.
- Sickle crises are precipitated by stresses such as infection, dehydration and hypoxia. Patients are likely to have an African, Middle Eastern or Mediterranean background (heterozygous individuals are resistant to malaria). Thrombotic presentations include: pulmonary syndrome, cerebral syndrome, bony crisis and avascular necrosis.
- Behçet's syndrome is identified by a history of orogenital ulceration and the presence of pathergy (the development of erythematous papules >2 mm in diameter at sites of skin trauma, e.g. injection sites).
- Antiphospholipid syndrome patients have a history of clots, miscarriage and a livedo reticularis type rash.

Note that homocystinuria can also cause both arterial and venous thrombosis.

Warfarin and heparin
Clotting factors II, VII, IX, X

Topic facts
The vitamin K-dependent clotting factors that warfarin inhibits are shown above.

- **Warfarin** – important facts:
  - extrinsic pathway
  - monitor with the INR (international normalized ratio) test
  - vitamin K-dependent pathway (vitamin K is a fat-soluble vitamin essential for the production of factors II, VII, IX and X; it enables the γ-carboxylation of the profactors to their active state)
  - the peak effect of warfarin occurs 48 h after ingestion
  - warfarin has an early prothrombotic effect action as a result of its effects on proteins C + S (the body's natural anticoagulants).

- **Heparin** – important facts:
  - intrinsic pathway
  - monitor with the APTT (activated partial thromboplastin time) test
  - heparin potentiates the action of anti-thrombin 3 (which in turn activates thrombin and clotting factors VIII, IX, XI and XII)
  - half-life 2 h
  - low-molecular-weight heparins do not prolong the APTT; they have a predictable anticoagulant effect and do not require monitoring unless in long-term use; in this case use the factor Xa assay to assess the degree of anticoagulation
  - heparin-induced thrombocytopenia (HIT) is an immune reaction; it occurs in 5 per cent of patients and presets with thrombosis. Platelet activating arhibodies cause platelets to clump. This causes simultaneous thrombosis and thrombocytopaenia.

Cardiology

- Atrial fibrillation (AF)
- Atrial septal defect (ASD)
- Bradycardia
- Cardiac apex
- Cardiac arrest
- Collapsing pulse
- Congenital heart disease
- Digoxin
- Eisenmenger's syndrome
- Endocarditis
- Extrasystoles
- Fallot's tetralogy
- Heart block
- Heart failure
- Hypertension
- Jugular venous pressure
- Kussmaul's sign
- Murmurs
  - Aortic regurgitation
  - Aortic stenosis
  - Mitral regurgitation
  - Mitral stenosis
- Myocardial infarction
- Prolonged Q–T interval
- Restrictive cardiomyopathy
  - Turner's syndrome

Atrial fibrillation (AF)
Heart/Lung/Hormones/Alcohol

Cardiology

Heart
Lone AF
Ischaemia
Rheumatic disease
Hypertension
Atrial sepral defect (ASD)
Pericarditis

Lung
Pneumonia
Pulmonary embolus
Chronic lung disease
Carcinoma

Hormones
Hyperthyroidism

Alcohol

Topic facts

The more common causes of AF are summarized above by category:
- AF is a common cardiac arrhythmia characterized by an irregular heart rate and the absence of visible 'p' waves on the ECG. It is common in elderly people and affects up to 10 per cent of those over the age of 80.
- AF is classified into permanent, persistent (but responsive to cardioversion) and paroxysmal types.
- Patients with paroxysmal AF are managed with β blockade and anticoagulation.
- Rate control is as important as rhythm control in prevention of cardiovascular events and stroke (β blockers have replaced digoxin as first-line treatment for persistent AF).
- Clinically AF is an irregularly irregular pulse varying in both rate and volume. Multiple ectopics can mimic AF, so an ECG is required to confirm the diagnosis.

Atrial septal defect (ASD)

QRS (refers to the QRS complex on an ECG)
Quiet systolic murmur
Right
- Axis
- Bundle-branch block
- Ventricular hypertrophy

Secundum

Topic facts

This topic aids recall of the clinical and ECG findings in patients with an ostium secundum ASD. Ostium primum ASDs have the same findings apart from axis deviation, which is to the left.

- ASDs are congenitally acquired defects of the atrial septum that allow blood flow between the left and right atria. They are common (>15 per cent of adults have an unfused foramen ovale through which a cardiac catheter can be passed from the right to left atrium).
- ASDs are labelled from the ventricle upwards.
- Low atrium – ostium primum.
- Mid-atrium – ostium secundum.
- Fixed splitting is characteristic of an ASD. This means that the second heart sound is split into its separate components (aortic and pulmonary valve closure) and that the time of the split is constant throughout inspiration and expiration. Normally, splitting varies with respiration because negative pressure in inspiration increases right ventricular volume, which delays pulmonary valve closure. In an ASD the extra blood is distributed equally between both sides, so the timing remains constant or 'fixed'.
- The heart valves of the second sound close in alphabetical order, i.e. **a**ortic first, **p**ulmonary second.
- Primum is associated with trisomy 21 (Down syndrome).
- Paradoxical emboli occur when clots pass through an ASD bypassing the lung to cause a stroke.

Bradycardia

Bradycardia **M**eans **A** **S**low **H**eart

  β **B**lockers

  Myocardial infarction

  Active individuals

  Sinoatrial disorder

  Hypothyroidism

Topic facts

Sinus bradycardia is defined as a heart rate <60 beats/min. The common causes are listed above.

- β Blockade is the most common cause of sinus bradycardia seen in hospital patients.
- Very fit individuals may have a slow resting heart rate.
- Heart block is suggested by a heart rate <40 beats/min. An ECG trace will show a dissociation between the 'p' waves and the QRS complexes. QRS complexes are broad because the focus is in the ventricles. Cannon waves (atrial contraction against a closed tricuspid valve) may be seen in complete heart block as a result of loss of synchronicity between atria and ventricles.
- Heart rate is the best clinical indicator of thyroid status (i.e. under-/over-active). Other indicators of thyroid status are:
  - tremor
  - sweaty palms
  - reflexes (test ankle)
  - AF
  - thyroid bruit
  - lid lag.

Candidates should be aware that most thyroid patients presented will be euthyroid. The presence of eye signs does not indicate hyperthyroidism – patients with Graves' disease may be hyper-, hypo- or euthyroid.

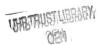

Cardiac apex
VT
   Volume overload
   Thrusting
pH
   Pressure overload
   Heaving

Topic facts
The correct terminology for the cardiac apex beat is summarized here to enable rapid recall.

- The cardiac apex is the most lateral and inferior point at which the cardiac pulsation is clearly palpable. In normal individuals this lies in the fifth intercostal space in the mid-clavicular line. If the cardiac apex is not palpable you must check for dextrocardia.
- VT (as in ventricular tachycardia) is the mnemonic for a volume-overloaded apex. In the clinical exam this should be described as thrusting in nature, and you would expect the apex to be displaced. Use this terminology for those patients with aortic regurgitation, mitral regurgitation and other causes of volume overload.
- pH (as in the measure of acidity) is the mnemonic for a pressure-overloaded apex. In the clinical exam this should be described as heaving in nature, and you would expect a non-displaced forceful apex. It may occur in cases of outflow obstruction such as aortic stenosis, coarctation of the aorta and hypertrophic cardiomyopathy.
- In many patients the apex is not easily palpable. This may be a result of either increased distance between the cardiac apex and chest wall (overweight patients, hyperinflated chest of chronic obstructive pulmonary disease or COPD) or other factors (pleural effusion, pericardial effusion, cardiomyopathy). If the apex is impalpable say so; this is a valid finding.

Cardiac arrest
Hs and Ts
Hypoxia
Hypovolaemia
Hypo-/hyperkalaemia
Hypothermia

Tension pneumothorax
Tamponade
Toxic/therapeutic disturbance
Thromboembolism

Topic facts
This topic covers the potentially reversible causes of a cardiac arrest, which need to be excluded during an acute event. It has been taken from the adult life support guidelines and should be familiar to all members of the on-call crash team.

- Hypoxia can be best assessed in the emergency situation by obtaining an arterial blood gas. This usually also provides a facility for rapid electrolyte analysis to identify hypo-/hyperkalaemia. Provide high-flow oxygen and protect the airway with the use of appropriate aids (nasopharyngeal, oropharyngeal or endotracheal airway).
- Hypothermia is defined as a core temperature of below 35°C. Patients at risk of hypothermia include elderly people, people who abuse alcohol, hypothyroid individuals and those with a history of exposure to cold (cold water, altitude). Look for ECG changes – J waves, and prolonged PR and QRS.

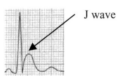 J wave

An ECG trace showing a J wave.

Collapsing pulse

A **C**ollapsing **P**ulse
Think **E**xercise **A**nd **P**regnancy

Independent

Aortic regurgitation
Cirrhosis
Patent ductus arteriosus

Hyperdynamic

Thyrotoxicosis
Exercise/**E**motion
Anaemia/**A**V (atrioventricular) fistula
Pregnancy/**P**yrexia

Topic facts

A collapsing pulse is defined as a large-volume pulse with a wide pulse pressure. The causes of a collapsing pulse can be divided into independent and hyperdynamic categories.

- Clinical features of a collapsing pulse:
  - large volume
  - tapping abrupt impulse
  - accentuation on elevating arm.
- To assess correctly for the presence of a collapsing pulse, place the palmar aspect of all four fingers across the radial pulse. Ask if the patient has pain in the shoulder. If not, proceed by raising the arm above the head, supporting the elbow. The character of the pulse changes on elevation to become a tapping abrupt impulse felt across all four fingers.
- There is a similar widening of the pulse pressure under the conditions of a hyperdynamic circulation. However, the collapsing nature may be less pronounced than independent causes.
- Look for associated clinical signs to identify the cause, e.g. early diastolic murmurs in aortic regurgitation, thyroid eye signs in hyperthyroid patients.

Congenital heart disease
Three holes
Three blocked tubes
Three blue babies

Three holes (left-to-right shunt)
ASD
Ventricular septal defect (VSD)
Patent ductus arteriosus

Three blocked tubes
Aortic stenosis
Pulmonary stenosis
Coarctation of the aorta

Three blue babies (right-to-left shunt)
Tetralogy of Fallot
Truncus arteriosus
Transposition of the great vessels

Topic facts
This well-known medical mnemonic lists the causes of congenital heart disease categorized by the direction of shunt and presence of 'holes':
- ASDs are the most common congenital heart disorders, and are discussed in more detail on page 20.
- VSDs are also common and account for up to a quarter of all congenital heart disease.
- VSDs may close spontaneously and management depends on size and symptoms. Small asymptomatic VSDs require no further intervention other than prophylaxis for subacute bacterial endocarditis (SBE). Symptomatic patients with moderate-to-large VSDs are at risk of developing Eisenmenger's syndrome (see page 27). Early surgical repair is necessary to prevent irreversible changes.
- Right-to-left shunts cause cyanotic congenital heart disease. Look for cyanosis and clubbing in the clinical case.
- Fallot's tetralogy is discussed on page 30.

Digoxin
Digoxin is a little QT

Topic facts
Digoxin causes shortening of the Q–T interval.

- Q–T interval is defined as the period from the start of the QRS complex to the end of the T wave. Q–T interval decreases as heart rate increases. QTc or corrected QT takes this into account by comparing the Q–T and R–R intervals to correct for rate.

- Normal Q–T interval duration is <0.44 seconds (two big squares plus one little square on the ECG).

- Most drugs with cardiotoxic effects lead to a lengthening of the Q–T interval, e.g. amiodarone, phenothiazine, probucol, quinidine and tetracycline. Digoxin is the exception and causes QT shortening (prolonged Q–T intervals are discussed on page 41).

- Digoxin therapy can lead to ECG changes such as the 'reversed tick' ST depression – this is not a sign of toxicity. Toxic patients develop arrhythmias, particularly atrioventricular (AV) block and gastrointestinal symptoms (nausea, vomiting, diarrhoea).

- Digoxin and verapamil are contraindicated in patients with Wolff–Parkinson–White syndrome. This is because they act as AV node blockers, thereby encouraging use of the accessory pathway. They are also contraindicated in patients with cardiac amyloid.

- Digoxin is cleared through the kidneys and should be used with caution in patients with renal impairment.

- Digoxin therapy can lead to yellow tinged vision (xanthopsia).

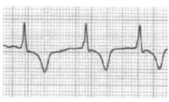

The reverse tick sign of digoxin therapy.

Eisenmenger's syndrome
Holes + Hypertension

Holes
ASD
VSD
Patent ductus arteriosus

Pulmonary hypertension

Topic facts
The causes of Eisenmenger's syndrome are summarized in this topic.
- Eisenmenger's syndrome is the onset of right ventricular hypertrophy, elevated right-sided pressures and pulmonary hypertension with the reversal of any left-to-right shunts.
- A large VSD is the most common cause, followed by pulmonary hypertension.
- Surgery can be performed to prevent Eisenmenger's syndrome developing, but intervention must be early because mortality from surgery is high once changes of Eisenmenger's syndrome are established.
- There are three key clinical findings:
  - cyanosis
  - clubbing
  - pulmonary hypertension:
    - loud pulmonary second sound
    - left parasternal heave
    - prominent 'a' wave in the JVP (jugular venous pressure).
- The most appropriate first-line investigations are transthoracic echocardiogram, ECG and chest radiograph.
- The echocardiogram and ECG will demonstrate right ventricular hypertrophy (sum of R in V1 and S in V5 >12 small squares) and the chest radiograph will demonstrate pulmonary hypertension (prominent vascular markings with peripheral pruning).

Endocarditis

Infected **V**alves **M**ean **E**ndocarditis

   Infective features:

      Malaise

      Fever

      Weight loss

   Vasculitis:

      Splinter haemorrhages: small infarcts seen in the nail

      Janeway lesions: palmar macules

      Osler's nodes: painful finger pulps

      Roth's spots: black spots found on the fundus

   Murmurs

   Emboli

Topic facts

The clinical findings of bacterial endocarditis are summarized here.

- Bacterial endocarditis is an infection of the heart valves. Left-sided valves are most commonly affected (the exception to this is intravenous drug abusers in whom 50 per cent develop tricuspid valve endocarditis).
- The most common organisms are *Streptococcus viridans* and *Staphylococcus aureus*.
- *Streptococcus bovis* endocarditis is associated with colon cancer and requires colonoscopy follow-up.
- Investigate with serial blood cultures taken from different venepuncture sites. These are vital and positive in the majority.
- If empirical treatment is required before blood culture results, use benzylpenicillin and gentamicin.
- Antibiotic therapy is required for 4–6 weeks.

Extrasystoles

Irregular **H**earts **A**re **D**angerous

Ischaemia/**I**diopathic
Hyperthyroid
Atrial enlargement
Digoxin

Topic facts

This topic lists common causes of extrasystoles.

- Extrasystolic beats may be premature or delayed (escape complexes). Premature beats occur earlier than one would expect compared with the regular rhythm. Escape beats occur later than expected and may be caused by a sick sinus node failing to fire as expected.

- Ectopic beats may be ventricular (broad complex) or supraventricular (narrow complex) in origin.

- Supraventricular ectopics can be atrial ('p' wave abnormal, absent or occurs after the QRS) or junctional (no P wave). The QRS complex is identical to that of sinus beats.

- Ventricular ectopics are easily identified because the morphology of the QRS complex differs from that of the normal complexes. Ventricular ectopics are common and most are not associated with morbidity.

- An alternating pattern of normal beat followed by ectopic beat is called bigeminy. This may be supraventricular or ventricular in origin and is associated with ischaemic heart disease. In some cases this can be identified clinically by palpation of the peripheral pulse, which alternates between large-volume and low-volume beats.

- R on T phenomenon is associated with ventricular fibrillation and death. It describes the situation where a ventricular ectopic complex occurs early in the T wave.

Fallot's tetralogy
ROPE

Right ventricular hypertrophy
Overriding aorta
Pulmonary stenosis
Extra hole (VSD)

Topic facts

The findings that make up Fallot's tetralogy are listed in this topic.

- Fallot's tetralogy is the most common cardiac cause of central cyanosis in a young patient. Most patients will have had surgical correction. It is likely to be present as a PACES case.
- Key clinical findings:
  - clubbing
  - central cyanosis
  - unilaterally weak radial pulse
  - midline thoracotomy scar
  - left parasternal heave (of right ventricular hypertrophy or RVH)
  - loud ejection systolic murmur.
- The weak unilateral radial pulse (usually the left) is a result of a Blalock shunt operation (part of a corrective surgical procedure). The shunt reduces blood flow to the radial artery.
- The ejection systolic murmur is the result of pulmonary stenosis. Right-sided murmurs are accentuated by asking the patient to inspire maximally.
- Investigation of Fallot's tetralogy (cardiac catheter) identifies:
  - VSD – right-to-left shunt (sats of left ventricle [LV] low)
  - pulmonary stenosis – pressure drop across the valve (>10 mmHg)
  - overriding aorta – aortic O_2 saturations < LV O_2 saturations (the right ventricle [RV] empties into the overriding aorta).

Heart block

Slow **R**ate **I**ndicates **D**amaged **C**onduction

    Stenosis (aortic)
    Rheumatic fever
    Infarcts/**I**schaemia
    Digoxin
    Congenital

Cardiology

Topic facts

The common causes of complete heart block are summarized in this mnemonic.

- Third-degree heart block is defined as the complete absence of AV conduction resulting in a ventricular escape rhythm.
- The heart rate is typically <40 beats/min. P waves may be present but there is no association between the 'p' waves and the QRS complex. QRS morphology is abnormal because the focus lies within the ventricle.
- Symptoms of heart block include lethargy, reduced exercise tolerance and syncope.
- Irregular cannon waves may be seen in the jugular vein as a result of loss of synchronicity between atria and ventricles. These are large 'a' waves resulting from atrial contractions against a closed tricuspid valve.
- The aortic valve lies adjacent to the AV junction, so disease affecting the aortic valve can lead to impairment of conduction. Aortic stenosis and complete heart block after aortic valve replacement surgery are examples of this.
- Drugs other than digoxin may cause AV blockade – common examples are β blockers and calcium channel blockers, e.g. verapamil.
- Management of complete heart block is by pacing. The patients to pace are those with: complete heart block, Möbitz type 2 blocks (2 : 1, 3 : 1), left anterior hemiblocks with syncopal attacks and sick sinus syndromes.

Heart failure

Heart failure + liver disease

Alcohol **S**trained **H**eart

   Alcohol/**A**myloid
   Sarcoid/**S**ystemic sclerosis
   Haemochromatosis

Heart failure + kidney failure

Sick **H**eart **A**nd **D**amaged **K**idney

   Systemic sclerosis
   Hypertension
   Amyloid
   Diabetes mellitus
   Kidney artery atherosclerosis

Heart failure + normal sized heart

Cardiac **F**ailure **N**o **C**ardiomegaly

   Constrictive pericarditis
   Flash pulmonary oedema
   Neurogenic pulmonary oedema
   Cardiomyopathy restrictive

Topic facts

There are many causes of heart failure. The differential diagnosis can be narrowed by identification of the presence of coexistent organ failure or heart failure in the absence of cardiomegaly. Three useful categories of heart failure are listed in this topic.

Hypertension
RACE
Renal diseases
Alcohol
Coarctation (of the aorta)
Endocrine

Topic facts
Primary (essential) hypertension accounts for 95 per cent of all cases of hypertension. Secondary causes account for the other 5 per cent of which renal diseases make up the majority (4 per cent).

This topic divides the causes of secondary hypertension into four categories. The endocrine causes of hypertension are summarized in the mnemonic below.

Endocrine causes of hypertension
RAMP
Renin (high levels):
- Renal artery stenosis
- Renin secreting tumours

Aldosterone:
- Adrenal adenoma (Conn's syndrome)
- Adrenal hyperplasia

Acromegaly
- Acromegaly (growth hormone excess)

Mineralocorticoid
- Cushing's syndrome (cortisol acts as a weak mineralocorticoid)

Phaeochromocytoma
- Catecholamine excess (epinephrine, norepinephrine)

Jugular venous pressure

Fluid **R**etention **C**auses **H**igh **V**enous **P**ressure

Fluid overload
Regurgitation (tricuspid)
Cor pulmonale
Heart block
Vena cava obstruction (superior)
Pericardial effusion/**P**ericarditis (constrictive)

Topic facts

This topic summarizes the causes of an elevated JVP.

- The JVP is a useful clinical tool that allows assessment of the right atrial pressure (because there are no valves between the right atrium and internal jugular).
- The JVP has a triphasic waveform made up of:
  a wave – **a**trial contraction
  c wave – **c**losure of tricuspid valve
  v wave – **v**entricular contraction.
- To assess the JVP the patient must be positioned correctly (45°). Measure the vertical height above the manubriosternal angle of the INTERNAL jugular vein. This runs from between the clavicular head and sternocleidomastoid to the ear lobe. Do not confuse JVP with the carotid pulsation. If unsure feel for the pulse – the jugular vein is easily occluded on palpation.
- Fixed elevation of the JVP indicates superior vena caval obstruction.
- Large v waves in time with the pulse shooting towards the ear lobe indicate tricuspid regurgitation. The liver may be pulsable and tender and the bilirubin may be raised (? icterus).
- Cannon waves are large 'a' waves. They occur when atria contract against a closed tricuspid valve as a result of loss of synchronicity between the atria and ventricles. They can be regular (nodal rhythm, ventricular tachycardia [VT]) or irregular (complete heart block, ventricular ectopics).

Kussmaul's sign

CPR

    Constrictive pericarditis

    Pericardial effusion

    Restrictive cardiomyopathy/**R**ight ventricular failure

Cardiology

Topic facts

Kussmaul's sign is defined as a rise in the JVP on inspiration. The causes are listed in the mnemonic.

- JVP normally falls on inspiration. This is because, in the normal individual, inspiration creates a negative pressure within the thoracic cavity. The same negative pressure that sucks air into the lungs also 'sucks' blood towards the heart, thus draining the jugular vein and lowering the JVP.

- In the three conditions listed the heart is unable to expand normally on filling. Sucking blood towards the heart on inspiration rapidly fills the small restricted/constricted ventricular cavity. The remainder overspills into the jugular vein, leading to the paradoxical rise in JVP.

- Common clinical presentations of constrictive and restrictive causes are reduced exercise tolerance, dyspnoea and oedema. A pericardial knock may be present.

- Echocardiography is the best first investigation to request in those with Kussmaul's sign. It will help differentiate between pericardial effusion and restrictive or constrictive causes. Also it is cheap, widely available, non-invasive and rapidly accessible.

- Restrictive and constrictive causes may be difficult to differentiate because the history, physical and echocardiographic findings may be very similar. Magnetic resonance imaging (MRI) is the investigation of choice because it allows the best assessment of pericardial involvement.

Murmurs

Aortic regurgitation

Aortic **R**egurg **C**auses **E**xtreme **B**reathlessness

Aortic dissection
Rheumatic fever
Congenital bicuspid valve
Endocarditis
Blood pressure (hypertension)

Topic facts

This mnemonic lists the common causes of aortic regurgitation. Rheumatic fever and infective endocarditis are the most common causes, followed by hypertension. Aortic regurgitation complicates several conditions; these are summarized in the mnemonic below.

Conditions associated with aortic regurgitation
MARS

Marfan's syndrome
Ankylosing spondylitis
Rheumatoid arthritis
Syphilis

- Aortic regurgitation is a common PACES case. The clinical findings are of a large-volume pulse, collapsing in nature, with a displaced apex.
- The apex is described as thrusting and is the result of volume overload. An early diastolic murmur is heard best down the left parasternal edge in inspiration, with the patient leaning forwards.
- Check for signs of the associated diseases. Ankylosing spondylitis is easy to miss in the patient lying on the bed. A useful trick is to ask the patient to move the head to enable you to assess the JVP. Ankylosing spondylitis patients will find this difficult.

Murmurs
Aortic stenosis

Really **B**ad **C**alcification
    Rheumatic heart disease
    Bicuspid aortic valve
    Calcified aortic valve

Topic facts

The common causes of aortic stenosis are listed in this topic in order of common occurrence.

- Aortic stenosis is a common PACES case and most candidates will correctly identify the diagnosis. In order to pass, the clinical examination and presentation need to be slick and include an assessment of severity.
- Clinical markers of severity in aortic stenosis:
  - slow rising pulse
  - narrow pulse pressure
  - quiet second heart sound.
- Amplitude of the murmur is not associated with severity. In critical aortic stenosis, the volume of flow may be so low that no murmur is audible.
- Clinical findings are of a small-volume pulse with a slow rising character. The apex is non-displaced and described as heaving as a result of the pressure loading. The second heart sound is (possibly) quiet and an ejection systolic murmur is heard in the second intercostal space in the aortic region. The murmur is loudest in expiration and classically radiates to the carotid arteries.
- As with all valvular disease, patients with aortic stenosis require endocarditis prophylaxis when undergoing dental or surgical procedures.
- ACE (angiotensin-converting enzyme) inhibitors and nitrates are relatively contraindicated in aortic stenosis.
- Aortic valve replacement should be offered to:
  - all symptomatic patients
  - aortic gradients >50 mmHg.

Murmurs
Mitral regurgitation

Mitral **R**egurg **D**amages **P**ump **F**unction

- **M**uscle damage (papillary)
- **R**heumatic fever
- **D**egenerative valve disease
- **P**rolapse
- **F**unctional regurgitation (LV dilatation)

Topic facts

This mnemonic lists the causes of mitral regurgitation. The most common cause is degenerative valve disease followed by rheumatic heart disease, functional regurgitation, prolapse and papillary muscle damage.

Causes of mitral valve prolapse
POEM plus

- **P**seudoxanthoma elasticum
- **O**steogenesis imperfecta
- **E**hlers–Danlos syndrome
- **M**arfan's syndrome

plus:

Congenital heart disease
Congestive cardiomyopathy
Polycystic kidney disease
Hypertrophic cardiomyopathy
Mitral valve surgery
Fabry's disease
Systemic lupus erythematosus (SLE)

- Clinical findings are of a displaced apex with a pansystolic murmur heard loudest in expiration at the apex and radiating to the axilla. (The murmur of prolapse is late systolic. Prolapse occurs in >5 per cent of the population)

Murmurs
Mitral stenosis
Rheumatic fever

Topic facts

Mitral stenosis is included for completeness as one of the four most commonly occurring murmurs at PACES. It is caused by rheumatic fever in the vast majority of cases. All other causes are extremely rare.

- Mitral stenosis is a narrowing of the mitral valve and develops 20–40 years after the initial episode of rheumatic fever. The normal mitral valve area is 4–6 cm^2, and stenosis is considered critical when the valve area is reduced to <1 cm^2.
- Clinical findings:
  - an irregularly irregular pulse (the majority are in AF)
  - a non-displaced tapping apex (palpable first heart sound)
  - loud first heart sound; then second heart sound followed by an opening snap and a mid-diastolic murmur (heard best with the patient in the left lateral position – this brings the mitral valve closer to the chest wall).
- If a patient has clinical findings but no audible murmur, the patient should be exercised to try to induce the murmur. After requesting the examiner's permission, ask the patient quickly to lean forward and touch his or her toes 10 times and then listen again.
- The sooner the opening snap occurs (after the second heart sound), the more severe the mitral stenosis.
- The main complications of mitral stenosis are heart failure, pulmonary hypertension, thrombotic emboli, endocarditis and pulmonary oedema.
- Management of mitral stenosis includes anticoagulation, rate control for those in AF and valve replacement for those with symptomatic disease.
- Valvotomy is possible in mobile, non-calcified valves.

Myocardial infarction (risk factors)

DB FAGS

Diabetes mellitus
Blood pressure
Family history/**F**ats
Age
Gender
Smoking

Previous heart attacks are an important risk factor not listed.

Topic facts

This topic lists the cardiovascular risk factors.

- Cardiovascular risk factors are a hot topic. They must be included as a risk assessment in a cardiovascular history case.
- Driving post-infarction is another important topic and is summarized as:
  - drivers must inform the DVLA after a myocardial infarction (MI)
  - drivers may resume driving a private vehicle 1 month after their MI if deemed fit
  - those with LGV/PCV (large goods vehicle/passenger-carrying vehicle) licences must complete three stages of the Bruce protocol off antianginals without evidence of ischaemia.

(The Driver and Vehicle Licensing Agency [DVLA] website provides up-to-date information on rules for driving in different medical conditions. MRCP candidates should read their guidelines on MI and fits. Drivers have a duty to disclose information to the DVLA and will not be insured if they fail to do so. Should a patient refuse to disclose to the DVLA, the doctor must warn the patient that he or she will be forced to disclose this information, because of a doctor's duty of care to protect the public. This measure is a last resort)

Prolonged Q–T interval (drug causes)

A **P**rolonged **Q–T**

  Amiodarone

  Phenothiazines/**P**robucol

  Quinine

  Tetracycline

Topic facts

The common drug causes of a prolonged Q–T interval are summarized in this mnemonic.

- Q–T interval is defined as the period from the start of the QRS complex to the end of the T wave. A normal Q–T interval duration is <0.44 seconds (two big squares and one little square on the ECG).
- Prolongation of the Q–T interval is associated with syncope and sudden death as a result of VT. Prolonged Q–T interval is particularly associated with a type of VT called torsades de pointes (also known as polymorphic VT).
- Non-drug causes of a prolonged Q–T interval include long QT syndrome (LQTS) and QT prolongation after an MI.
- LQTS is caused by a transmembrane ion channel defect. It is inherited as autosomal dominant in most patients. LQTS is a cause of sudden death (especially if there is a family history of this).
- The treatment of a prolonged Q–T interval depends on whether the disorder is acquired or congenital.
  - **a**cquired – **a**ccelerate
  - **c**ongenital – **s**low down.
- Acquired QT prolongation is managed by overdrive pacing or using isoprenaline.
- Congenital QT prolongation is treated with β blockade and implantable defibrillators in those with persistent arrhythmias.

Torsades de pointes (Sinusoidal pattern outlined)

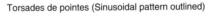

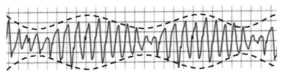

Restrictive cardiomyopathy

Amyloid **D**eposits **C**an **S**top **H**eart **E**xpansion

Amyloid
Drugs
Carcinoid
Sarcoid/Systemic fibrosis
Haemochromatosis
Endomyocardial fibrosis

Topic facts

This topic lists the more common causes of restrictive cardiomyopathy.

- Restrictive cardiomyopathy is a disease in which the ventricles become stiff and unable to expand fully.
- Infiltrative processes such as systemic sclerosis, amyloid, sarcoid and haemochromatosis are often implicated, although in some cases no underlying cause is found.
- Symptoms and signs are similar to constrictive pericarditis.
- Patients present with features of heart failure but on examination and investigation the heart is of a normal size.
- Kussmaul's sign – elevation of the JVP in inspiration may be present.
- Normally JVP falls on inspiration as negative pressure within the chest cavity sucks blood into the ventricles, thus emptying the jugular vein.
- In restrictive cardiomyopathy the ventricles cannot expand to accommodate the influx of blood and the overspill fills the jugular vein – hence the paradoxical rise in JVP.
- Investigation is with echocardiography and endomyocardial biopsy.
- Chemotherapy agents are associated with restrictive cardiomyopathy (doxyrubicin, 5-fluorouracil or 5-FU).

Turner's syndrome (cardiac findings)
Holes and Narrowings

Holes
ASD
VSD

Narrowings
Coarctation of the aorta
Aortic stenosis

Topic facts
The common congenital cardiac abnormalities associated with Turner syndrome are summarized in this topic.
- Turner syndrome (45 XO) is a genetic disorder associated with characteristic phenotypic appearances and cardiovascular abnormalities.
- Phenotypic features:
  - short stature
  - high-arched palate
  - webbed neck
  - cubitus valgus (wide carrying angle; this is demonstrated by asking the patient to hold the arms straight out in front with palms facing upwards; the forearm is seen to deviate laterally away from the elbow joint)
  - widely spaced nipples
  - short fourth metacarpals (these can be easily missed; ask the patient to make a fist, which makes the knuckles become more prominent; the fourth knuckle is recessed as a result of the shortened metacarpal)
  - low hairline.
- Amenorrhoea is a common mode of presentation.
- X-linked recessive conditions may present as full-blown conditions in Turner's syndrome due to the single X chromosome.
- Other congenital abnormalities in Turner's syndrome:
  - horseshoe kidney
  - streak ovaries
  - strabismus.

Cardiology

Neurology

- Altitudinal hemianopia
- Argyll Robertson pupil
- Autonomic neuropathy
- Bitemporal hemianopia
- Blackouts – syncope
- Bulbar palsy
- Carpal tunnel syndrome
- Central retinal vein occlusion
- Central scotoma
- Cerebellar signs
- Charcot joints
- Chorea
- Collapse on a psychiatric ward
- Coma
- Cranial nerves
- Dementia
- Dorsal columns
- Dysphasia
- Friedreich's ataxia
- Headache
- Horner's syndrome
- Impaired consciousness – alcohol abusers
- Mixed motor signs from the spinal cord
- Mononeuritis multiplex
- Optic atrophy
- Papilloedema
- Paraplegia/Tetraplegia
- Peripheral neuropathy
- Proximal myopathy
- Ptosis
- Retinitis pigmentosa
- Sensory ataxia

- Sixth nerve palsy
- Spastic paraparesis
- Stroke
- Tardive dyskinesia
- Third nerve palsy
- Tunnel vision
- Wasting of small muscles of the hand

Altitudinal hemianopia
Retina/Nerve/Cortex

Retina
Occlusions (branch retinal artery/vein)

Nerve (optic nerve)
Ischaemic optic neuropathy
Papilloedema

Cortex
Temporal lobe lesion
Parietal lobe lesion
Occipital lobe

Topic facts
Altitudinal hemianopia is the loss of either the upper or the lower half of the visual field. The causes of altitudinal hemianopia have been simplified here and are summarized into retina, nerve and cortex categories.

- Branch retinal artery occlusions are most commonly secondary to emboli. Patients complain of sudden, unilateral, painless, visual loss. Risk factors are the same as for cardiovascular disease. Rarer causes include vasculitis and thrombophilic states.
- Branch retinal vein occlusion presents similarly to branch retinal artery occlusion. Most cases are idiopathic but there is an association with thrombophilic states.
- Ischaemic optic neuropathy presents with altitudinal hemianopia (more commonly inferior), a relative afferent papillary defect and a pale swollen optic disc. It is associated with hypertension, diabetes and temporal arteritis.
- Pressure on the optic chiasm superiorly from anterior communicating artery aneurysms can also cause an altitudinal visual field defect.
- Lesions of the cortex can cause altitudinal visual loss.

Argyll Robertson pupil

'An Argyll Robertson pupil is like a prostitute, it accommodates but does not respond!' (to light).

Topic facts

This well-known medical mnemonic summarizes the clinical findings of Argyll Robertson pupils.

- Argyll Robertson pupils are small, irregular pupils, which constrict to accommodation but do not respond to light.
- The causes are:
  - syphilis
  - diabetes mellitus.
- Argyll Robertson pupils may become dilated in chronic cases. Candidates should then rely on the presence of pupil irregularity and associated clinical findings of syphilis or diabetes.
- Associated clinical findings of syphilis:
  - proprioception impaired (stamping ataxic gait and Romberg's test positive)
  - Charcot joints (typically the knee)
  - mixed motor signs from the spinal cord (absent reflexes with an upgoing plantar response)
  - aortic regurgitation.
- Associated findings of diabetes mellitus:
  - evidence of fingerpricks from blood sugar testing
  - peripheral vascular disease (shiny, cold, hairless legs with absent peripheral pulses)
  - neuropathy (sensory ataxia)
  - retinopathy (note use of thick glasses, white stick).

Autonomic neuropathy

Start **W**ith **P**rimary
Don't **F**orget **G**uillain–Barré syndrome

Primary (central)

Syringomyelia/**S**yringobulbia
Wernicke's encephalopathy
Primary selective autonomic failure (Riley–Day syndrome)/**P**arkinson's
   disease (Shy–Drager syndrome)

Peripheral

Diabetes mellitus
Familial dysautonomia/Familial amyloidosis
Guillain–Barré syndrome

Topic facts

Autonomic neuropathies are a group of disorders that impair the function
of the autonomic nervous system. They can be categorized into primary
(central) and peripheral causes.

- Both sympathetic and parasympathetic nervous systems are affected by
  the autonomic neuropathies.
- There are three main types of autonomic dysfunction:
  - gastrointestinal: gastroparesis, episodic nocturnal diarrhoea and colonic
    dilatation
  - cardiovascular: postural hypotension, elevated resting heart rate and
    loss of sinus arrhythmia
  - genitourinary: large residual volumes, retrograde ejaculation and
    impotence.
- Other causes of peripheral autonomic neuropathy include tabes dorsalis,
  alcohol-related neuropathy and Eaton–Lambert syndrome.

Bitemporal hemianopia

Pituitary **C**ompression **A**ffects **S**ight

    Pituitary tumour

    Craniopharyngioma

    Aneurysm

    Suprasellar meningioma

Topic facts

Bitemporal hemianopia is the loss of the lateral visual field bilaterally and is caused by compression of the optic chiasm. This topic lists the causes of bitemporal hemianopia in order of the most common occurrence.

- Pituitary tumours are divided into microadenomas (<1 cm) and macroadenomas (>1 cm). The latter may cause chiasmal compression.
- Craniopharyngioma is a slow-growing cystic tumour that can be found at any age. It commonly presents with headache, endocrine dysfunction (especially hypothyroidism) and visual field defects.
- Examine for features of endocrine gland hypo-/hyperfunction:
  - hypothyroidism
  - acromegaly
  - Cushing's disease
  - hypopituitarism.
- The examination sheet may provide a clue to the diagnosis such as 'this man complains of bumping into objects; please examine as you feel appropriate'.
- Bitemporal hemianopia can be incongruous (i.e. worse on one side than the other). Examine the fields carefully to differentiate between an incongruous bitemporal hemianopia and a unilateral visual field loss due to a lesion between the retina and the optic chiasm.
- Optic chiasm compression is investigated best by magnetic resonance imaging (MRI).

Blackouts – syncope

Always **E**xclude **V**asovagal **S**yncope

    Arrhythmia

    Epilepsy

    Vasovagal syncope

    Situational syncope

Topic facts

The common causes of transient loss of consciousness are summarized here.

- Syncope is a common presenting complaint on acute medical wards, and in the MRCP. Careful attention to history is important in determining the cause.

- Arrhythmias may be tachyarrhythmias or bradyarrhythmias. Look for a history of cardiovascular risk factors and cardiac disease. Symptoms such as palpitations, chest pain, shortness of breath and lack of warning before onset of syncope are consistent with a cardiac arrhythmia.

- Along with the arrhythmias category, consider other cardiac causes of syncope such as outflow obstruction (aortic stenosis, hypertrophic cardiomyopathy).

- Epilepsy is suggested if the syncope is associated with a history of witnessed tonic–clonic activity, pre-syncopal aura, a post-ictal period, loss of bladder control or injury (tongue biting, bruising).

- Vasovagal syncope is common in young adults. Symptoms of nausea, sweating, dizziness and light-headedness predominate. The episode may be precipitated by strong emotion or sensation, e.g. fear, pain.

- Situational syncope attacks are similar to vasovagal ones but are precipitated by specific situations such as micturation, defaecation and carotid sinus sensitivity.

- Initial investigations to request – ECG, postural blood pressure, blood glucose (? hypoglycaemia) ± chest radiograph.

Bulbar palsy
Bulbar palsy (LMN)
Bulbar **P**alsy **G**ets **M**outh
> **B**rain-stem tumour/**B**ulbia (syringo)
> **P**olio
> **G**uillain–Barré syndrome
> **M**otor neurone disease (MND)

Pseudobulbar palsy (UMN)
May **M**ean **S**troke
> **M**ultiple sclerosis (MS)
> **M**ND
> **S**troke

Topic facts
Bulbar palsy and pseudobulbar palsy are motor neuron lesions and present clinically with dysarthria. The more common causes are summarized above.

- Bulbar (refers to the medulla oblongata) palsy is a lower motor neurone (LMN) lesion resulting from damage of the cranial nerve nuclei in the medulla oblongata. MND is the most common cause.
- Pseudobulbar palsy is an upper motor neuron (UMN) lesion that results from damage to the corticobulbar tracts (these join the cranial nerve nuclei and brain cortex). Cerebrovascular accident (CVA) is the more common cause.
- Remember MND can affect both UMNs and LMNs and can cause either presentation.
- Bulbar palsy patients have a flaccid, wasted, fasciculating tongue and there may be impairment of chewing or swallowing.
- Pseudobulbar patients have a tight spastic tongue that the patient finds difficult to protrude. An exaggerated jaw jerk is present.

Carpal tunnel syndrome

TRAP

Thyroid

Rheumatoid arthritis

Acromegaly

Pregnancy/**P**ill

Topic facts

Carpal tunnel syndrome (CTS) is a disorder of nerve compression caused by the entrapment of the median nerve within the confined space of the carpal tunnel. This mnemonic summarizes the common causes.

- CTS may be precipitated by conditions causing soft tissue swelling such as pregnancy (fluid retention), acromegaly (continued growth of soft tissues) and hypothyroidism.
- β_2-Microglobulin deposition (a form of amyloid), found in rheumatoid arthritis, can lead to CTS.
- CTS is associated with manual jobs involving repetitive actions such as typing or sewing.
- Clinical presentation is of paraesthaesiae in a median nerve distribution (palmar aspect of the thumb and first two digits), which is typically worse at night and may radiate into the arm. Patients may complain of dropping objects or loss of power.
- Examine for evidence of thenar wasting and reduced power (thumb abduction and pinch grip). Tinel's test (tapping over the wrist) and Phalen's sign (hyperflexion of the wrist) are unreliable.
- Investigate with nerve conduction studies to help confirm diagnosis and assess severity. In patients with a strongly suggestive history but normal nerve conduction study, MRI may be considered.
- Management options consist of splinting, rest and non-steroidal anti-inflammatory drugs (NSAIDs), with surgical release for those with persistent symptoms.

Neurology

Central retinal vein occlusion

Fats **D**amage **B**ig **V**ein

Fats
Diabetes mellitus
Blood pressure
Viscosity (hyper-)

Topic facts

The common causes of central retinal vein occlusion are summarized in this topic.

- Central retinal vein occlusion is associated with hyperlipidaemia, diabetes mellitus, hypertension and hyperviscosity states such as myeloma, Waldenström's macroglobulinaemia, polycythaemia rubra vera and connective tissue disease.
- There is a characteristic sunray appearance seen on fundoscopy, with red streaks radiating like spokes from the central disc.
- Any visible veins are dilated and tortuous.
- Flame haemorrhages can be seen in the area drained by the vein. Cotton-wool spots may be present.
- Visual loss is incomplete and may occur suddenly or over a period of days and weeks.
- New vessel formation on the iris can occur later in presentation and lead to secondary glaucoma.
- Neovascularization can also occur near the optic disc and is a marker of retinal ischaemia. These patients are at risk of vitreous haemorrhage.
- First-line investigations should include erythrocyte sedimentation rate (ESR), serum glucose, lipid profile, serum electrophoresis and slit-lamp examination.
- Laser photocoagulation is the treatment of choice (panretinal photocoagulation).
- Post-occlusion follow-up is required along with secondary prevention to reduce the risk factors. Strict hypertension, lipid and glycaemic control are needed.

Neurology

Central scotoma

Middle **O**f **P**icture **R**uined
 Macular degeneration
 Optic atrophy
 Papilloedema/**P**apillitis
 Retrobulbar neuritis

Topic facts

Central scotoma is the loss of the central visual field. The most common causes are macular degeneration, optic atrophy, papilloedema/papillitis and retrobulbar neuritis.

- Age-related macular degeneration is the most common cause of progressive visual field loss in the UK. Fundoscopic findings of drusen suggest macular degeneration.
- Optic atrophy is the common end-finding of many different causes of optic nerve injury.
- The most common causes of optic atrophy are demyelination (MS), optic nerve compression and retinal artery occlusion.
- Retrobulbar neuritis is a neuritis localized to the optic nerve distal to the optic disc. Hence the optic disc appearance is unchanged; it is often said that 'the patient can see nothing and the doctor can see nothing'.
- Movement of the eye in retrobulbar neuritis is typically painful as a result of the muscles compressing the swollen nerve on change of gaze.
- Papilloedema is swelling of the optic disc secondary to raised intracranial pressure. Papillitis is swelling of the optic disc due to other causes. The fundus changes are the same.
- Papillitis is caused by optic neuritis, accelerated hypertension and retinal vein obstruction.
- MS causes both optic atrophy and retrobulbar optic neuritis.

Cerebellar signs

Major **B**alance **P**roblem **A**ffects **F**unction

Multiple sclerosis

Brain-stem vascular lesion

Posterior fossa space-occupying lesion/**P**araneoplastic syndrome

Alcohol cerebellar degeneration

Friedreich's ataxia

Topic facts

This mnemonic lists the causes of cerebellar signs in order of the most common occurrence in the UK (Balance refers to atopia).

- The cerebellar signs are:
  - dysdiadochokinesis (impaired rapid repetitive movements)
  - finger–nose pointing
  - nystagmus (fast phase towards the side of the lesion)
  - internuculear ophthalmoplegia (inability of the AD-ducting eye to follow the AB-ducting eye to maintain conjugate gaze due to a lesion in the medial longitudinal fasciculus)
  - ataxia (impaired balance: broad-based gait with impaired heel-to-toe walking)
  - intention tremor
  - staccato/scanning speech
  - hypotonic reflexes.
- Patients with subtle internuclear ophthalmoplegia can be best demonstrated by examining circades. Hold up a fist in one hand and a finger in the other. Ask the patient to look alternately between fist and finger. Look for slowing of the AD-ducting eye on repetitive movement.

Charcot joints

Look **S**everely **D**amaged

Leprosy
Syringomyelia/**S**yphilis
Diabetes mellitus

Sites

Elbow/shoulder: syringomyelia
Hips/knees: syphilis (tabes dorsalis)
Ankles/toes: diabetes mellitus.

Topic facts

Charcot joint or neuropathic arthropathy is a condition characterized by the progressive destruction of a joint as the result of recurrent trauma secondary to loss of joint sensation. This topic covers the causes of Charcot joints and sites affected.

- Charcot joints result in a grossly deformed but relatively pain-free joint (in comparison to the degree of joint destruction).
- The most common cause of Charcot joints is diabetes-related neuropathy and the most common joints affected are the ankle, tarsal and metatarsal joints.
- Syringomyelia is suggested by the presence of wasting in the hands with dissociated sensory loss.
- The management aim is to reduce stresses on the affected joint. Options include weight loss, use of walking aids (crutches, patellar tendon-bearing braces) and customized footwear. Surgery is possible in a few selected cases, but healing is often prolonged as a result of the underlying disease process.
- Complications of Charcot joint include ulceration over sites of bony protuberance and infection, including osteomyelitis.

Chorea

I Have **A F**rustrating **M**ovement **D**isorder

Infections
- Sydenham's chorea
- Encephalitis

Haematological
- Polycythaemia rubra vera

Autoimmune
- Lupus erythematosus

Familial
- Huntington's disease
- Wilson's disease
- Ataxia telangiectasia

Metabolic and endocrine
- Chorea gravidarum (chorea of pregnancy)
- Thyrotoxicosis

Drugs **(LOP)**
- Levodopa
- Oestrogen
- Phenytoin

Topic facts

Chorea is characterized by excessive, non-repetitive, irregular, abrupt, jerky movements. This complex movement disorder has many causes that are split into categories here to aid recall.

- Drug-induced chorea (levadopa) is one of the most common causes seen.
- Huntington's disease occurs between ages 35–50, often accompanied by dementia.
- Senile chorea also exists and is idiopathic.

Neurology

Collapse on a psychiatric ward
FLAT

Fits

Long QT

Acute intermittent porphyria

Tricyclic antidepressant overdose

Topic facts

This mnemonic lists causes of collapse specific to psychiatric admissions.

- Fits on the psychiatric ward may be caused by alcohol withdrawal, drug abuse or epilepsy. (There is an association between epilepsy and schizophrenia.)
- QT prolongation can be caused by common psychiatric agents such as the antipsychotics (chlorpromazine, haloperidol, mesoridazine, quetiapine and thioridazine) and antidepressants (fluoxetine, paroxetine and venlafaxine). Prolonged Q–T interval is associated with cardiac arrhythmias and syncope (see page 41).
- Acute intermittent porphyria (AIP) is an autosomal dominant disorder that results from porphobilinogen deaminase dysfunction. This leads to a build-up of the harmful porphyrin pathway precursors (aminolaevulanic acid and porphobilinogen). The defective genes are found on chromosome 11.
  - Typical features include hypertension, tachycardia, nausea and vomiting, constipation, and neurological manifestations including psychosis, motor neuropathy and, when very aggressive, seizures.
  - Precipitants of attacks include many drugs, alcohol, fasting and infection.
  - Management includes withdrawal of precipitants, high calorie diet (reduces precursors of haem synthesis through enzyme inhibition) and haem arginate infusion (inhibits porphyrin pathway through negative feedback).
  - Give chlormethiazole for fits, a safe drug in AIP.

Coma

Mostly **D**ue **T**o **B**rain **E**ffects

Metabolic

- Electrolyte disturbance (glucose, sodium, calcium)
- Organ failure (renal, liver, lung with CO_2 retention)

Diffuse

- Brain hypoxia/ischaemia
- Encephalitis
- Hypertensive encephalopathy

Toxins

- Alcohol, carbon monoxide, sedative drugs

Brain cortex

- Tumour
- Trauma
- Infarct/bleed
- Demyelination

Endocrine

- Hypoadrenalism, hypothyroidism

Topic facts

The causes of impaired level of consciousness are summarized above into five categories.

- Electrolyte disturbance is a common finding especially in patients on diuretic therapy. Rapid correction can be dangerous, particularly in hyponatraemia. A rapid rise in serum osmolality may lead to shrinkage of the brain cells and death (central pontine myelinolysis). Fluid is restricted to 500–1500 mL and the aim is to raise serum sodium gradually.

Neurology

Cranial nerves

Oh **O**h **O**h **T**o **T**ouch **A**nd **F**eel.
Very **G**ood **V**eal **A**nd **H**am

  Olfactory
  Optic
  Oculomotor
  Trochlear
  Trigeminal
  Abducens
  Facial
  Vestibulocochlear
  Glossopharyngeal
  Vagus
  Accessory
  Hypoglossal

Topic facts

The twelve cranial nerves are summarized above in an adaptation of a well-known medical school mnemonic that is unpublishable!

- The cranial nerves can be divided anatomically into three groups of four. The first four originate in the midbrain, the middle four in the pons and the last four in the medulla.
- The cranial nerves lie sequentially, with the first nerve found most anteriorly in the brain and the twelfth most posteriorly.
- There are important connections between the cranial nerves. An example of this is the medial longitudinal fasciculus, which connects the third and sixth cranial nerves. The sixth nerve must tell the third nerve when it is abducting the eye so that the contralateral eye can adduct and maintain conjugate gaze.
- MRCP candidates need to know the different causes of cranial nerve palsies.

Dementia
DEMENTIA PH
Drink (Wernicke–Korsakoff syndrome)

Encephalopathy

Multi-infarct

Normal pressure hydrocephalus

Thyroid (hypo)

Infection (HIV, Creutzfeldt–Jakob disease [CJD], syphilis)/**I**ntracerebral
bleed

Alzheimer's disease

Parkinson's disease

Huntington's disease

Topic facts
Dementia is an impairment of cognitive functioning (memory, behaviour
and reasoning) to such a degree that it impacts on an individual's normal
daily activities. The causes of dementia are summarized in this mnemonic.

- In most cases of dementia there is a progressive decline. It is important
  not to miss the potentially reversible causes such as hypothyroidism,
  encephalopathy and normal pressure hydrocephalus.
- Normal pressure hydrocephalus presents with the triad of gait dyspraxia,
  cognitive impairment and urinary incontinence. The gait is typically wide
  and shuffling and may be confused for parkinsonism.
- Korsakoff's syndrome presents with memory loss but otherwise well-
  preserved cognitive function. Characteristic findings are a retrograde
  amnesia, loss of insight, confabulation and difficulty in assimilating new
  information.
- Wernicke's encephalopathy (ophthalmoplegia, ataxia and confusion) may
  precede Korsakoff's syndrome.
- Both Wernicke's and Korsakoff's syndromes are caused by vitamin B_1
  deficiency as a result of alcohol abuse.
- Check thyroid-stimulating hormone (TSH) for hypothyroidism in all
  dementias.

Dorsal columns

VPL

Vibration
Proprioception
Light touch

Topic facts

The sensory modalities transmitted via the dorsal columns are covered in this topic.

- The sensory system is divided into two spinal tracts: the dorsal columns and the spinothalamic tract.
- The dorsal column carries vibration, proprioception and light touch fibres. Of these the most discriminatory is vibration, followed by proprioception and light touch.
- The spinothalamic tract carries sensory fibres for pain, temperature and crude touch. Pain is the most discriminatory of these.
- You will be expected to examine all modes of sensation during the clinical exam if asked for a neurological examination of a limb. A useful technique is to pay careful attention to the most discriminatory findings (i.e. vibration for dorsal columns and pain for spinothalamic tract) and ignore the other tests (proprioception, temperature, etc.), which are less reliable. Use the time going through the motions of the 'unreliable tests' to gather your thoughts as to the possible diagnosis and differential, so that you are ready to present as soon as you stop examining. However, because of a dissociated sensory loss.
- Differentiate between polyneuropathy ('glove-and-stocking') sensory loss and a dermatomal distribution of sensory deficit.
- Sensory loss may be complete or dissociated (unequal loss of sensory modalities). Dissociated loss occurs in cord disease, syringomyelia, Brown–Séquard disease and tabes dorsalis.

Dysphasia

Broca's area: **FIG**
Wernicke's area: **STiG**

Broca's area

Frontal **I**nferior **G**yrus

Wernicke's area

Superior **T**emporal **G**yrus

Topic facts

Knowledge of the anatomical localization of the speech centres is important in localization of pathology. These memory aids help rapid recall.

- Broca's area is found in the frontal inferior gyrus or FIG. A lesion affecting Broca's area leads to non-fluent speech with preserved comprehension and loss of prosody (the natural melodic sound of speech). This is often termed an 'expressive dysphasia'.
- Broca's area is associated with a hemiplegia.
- Wernicke's area is found in the superior temporal gyrus or STiG. Lesions in this area lead to a fluent unintelligible speech with loss of comprehension. This is often termed a 'receptive dysphasia'.
- Wernicke's area is associated with visual field deficits.
- Both areas may be affected, leading to global dysphasia with loss of fluency and comprehension.
- Examination of speech should include an assessment of:
  - articulation ('British constitution', 'baby hippopotamus')
  - repetition
  - comprehension ('shut your eyes')
  - nominal dysphasia (pen, watch, keys)
  - higher mental function.
- Cerebrovascular accidents are the most common cause of dysphasia.

Neurology

Friedreich's ataxia

DOC

Diabetes

Optic atrophy

Cardiomyopathy

Topic facts

Friedreich's ataxia is an autosomal recessive, trinucleotide repeat disorder. This mnemonic summarizes the common associated findings of Friedreich's ataxia.

- Friedreich's ataxia is characterized by the triad of:
  - skeletal deformity:
    - pes cavus
    - scoliosis
  - cerebellar signs:
    - intention tremor
    - cerebellar dysarthria
    - dysdiadochokinesis
    - cerebellar ataxia
  - mixed motor signs:
    - extensor plantar response
    - absent ankle and knee reflexes.
- The abnormal trinucleotide repeat is GAA and it is located on the long arm of chromosome 9.
- Anticipation is a phenomenon found in trinucleotide repeat disorders. As the repeat is passed on from one generation to the next, the sequence expands in length. This results in earlier onset of symptoms and increasing severity of disease.
- Peripheral neuropathy (predominantly sensory) is a common finding in patients with Friedreich's ataxia.
- The most common presenting features are gait ataxia, intention tremor and cerebellar speech.

Headache

Migraine **C**auses **V**ery **S**evere **H**eadache

Migraine/**M**eningitis

Cluster and tension/**C**hronic raised intracranial pressure (ICP)

Vasculitis

Space-occupying lesion

Haemorrhage (subarachnoid haemorrhage or SAH)

Topic facts

The differential diagnosis of headache is covered here.

- History is critical in identifying the precipitating cause.
- Tension headaches are typically bilateral and felt as a diffuse band around the head or weight on top of the head. Tender spots are often present.
- Cluster headaches often present with a headache plus epiphoria (a watery eye). There may be recurrence of headache over a period of weeks and months followed by a lengthy remission.
- Migrainous headache classically presents with an aura including visual disturbances and transient dysarthria. There may be vasomotor disturbances including flushing and pallor. Severe headache with photophobia follows. Migraine can occur without aura.
- Patients with chronic raised ICP present with headaches, diplopia, nausea and vomiting, and sixth nerve palsies. Fundal examination reveals papilloedema. There is a compensatory elevation in blood pressure and a decrease in heart rate.
- Benign intracranial hypertension is a type of chronic raised ICP typically found in young, adult, overweight women. Treatment is with bendrofluazide and lumbar puncture.

Horner's syndrome
ABC SPLIT
Aneurysms
Brain-stem vascular disease
Carotid dissection

Syringomyelia
Pancoast's tumour
Lymphadenopathy (cervical)
Idiopathic
Trauma and surgery

Topic facts
Horner's syndrome is caused by a lesion of the sympathetic nervous system. The sympathetic chain runs through the midbrain, medulla and spinal cord, exiting at T1–2. It then ascends through the chest via the lung apex and carotid artery. Causes of lesions along this pathway are summarized in this topic.

- Horner's syndrome consists of the triad:
  - miosis (constricted pupil)
  - ptosis (drooping eyelid)
  - anhidrosis (loss of sweating).
- These features may be recalled by remembering the actions of the sympathetic nerve during a stress situation such as being attacked. Pupils dilate to allow best possible vision for escape, eyes open wide and the individual sweats with fear. Loss of sympathetic innervation therefore leads to the reverse.
- The most common cause is trauma and surgery followed by aneurysms and brain-stem vascular disease.
- Horners syndrome may be the only manifestation of carotid dissection. In a newly presenting Horner's syndrome of uncertain cause an urgent carotid and head MRI should be performed.
- On clinical examination, it is important to identify whether the abnormal pupil is the small or large one. Watching response to direct and consensual light reflex tests this best.
- A Horner's syndrome pupil is small and fixed, i.e. does not respond well to direct light. The contralateral pupil constricts normally to light.

Impaired consciousness – alcohol abusers

Boozers **F**all **I**nto **T**he **E**mpty **G**utter

    Brain bleed (subdural)

    Fits (withdrawal/epileptic)

    Infection (TB, meningitis)

    Trauma

    Encephalopathy (hepatic/Wernicke's encephalopathy)

    Gastrointestinal bleed

Topic facts

Potential causes of impaired consciousness in patients with chronic alcohol abuse are summarized here.

- Alcohol abusers are vulnerable individuals and frequent attendees at hospital. It is important that impaired conscious levels are appropriately assessed even if the patient is a recurrent attendee. Assumption of alcohol intoxication as the causal factor puts both you and your patient at risk.

- Alcohol-dependent patients are at high risk of subdural haematomas (SDHs) because of their tendency to fall and their impaired coagulation. Acute SDHs have evidence of head trauma clinically, but in chronic SDHs this may be absent. A high index of suspicion and evidence of raised ICP is needed to make the diagnosis.

- Fits may be the result of alcohol withdrawal (in which case use a reducing-dose chlordiazepoxide regimen), or epilepsy due to lowering of seizure threshold.

- Alcohol, homelessness and malnutrition are independent risk factors associated with active tuberculosis (TB) infection.

- Trauma may be the result of falls or assaults, both of which are more common in alcohol-dependent patients.

- Encephalopathy may be a result of decompensated liver disease (hepatic) or vitamin B_1 (thiamine) deficiency (Wernicke's encephalopathy – ophthalmoplegia, ataxia, confusion).

Mixed motor signs from the spinal cord

Mixed **S**igns **F**rom **T**he **C**ord

   MND

   Subacute combined degeneration

   Friedreich's ataxia

   Taboparesis (syphilis)

   Conus medilaris compression

Topic facts

'Mixed motor neuron signs' means that a combination of both UMN and LMN signs is present. A typical combination would be upgoing plantars with absent knee and ankle reflexes. The differential diagnosis is listed here.

- UMN signs:
  - increased tone
  - clonus
  - hyperreflexia
  - upgoing plantars.
- LMN signs:
  - fasciculation
  - muscle wasting
  - hypotonia
  - reduced/absent reflexes.
- Patients with conus medilaris compression will have signs limited to the lower limbs. Candidates often confuse the conus medilaris and the cauda equina. The cauda equina involves only LMNs because it lies below the end of the spinal cord. The conus medilaris contains the tapering end of the spinal cord and the LMN fibres that have left the cord at higher levels. Thus, conus medilaris lesions have mixed motor neuron signs.
- Subacute combined degeneration is common; look for dorsal column signs (see page 62).

Mononeuritis multiplex
DC SLAC
Diabetes mellitus
Connective tissue disease (see page 162)

Sarcoid
Lyme disease
Amyloid
Carcinoma

Topic facts
Mononeuritis multiplex is a group of disorders that can cause both motor and sensory peripheral neuropathies, typically affecting several nerve areas. The causes of mononeuritis multiplex are summarized above.

- Mononeuritis multiplex is the most common cause of a sixth nerve palsy, and the second most common cause of a third nerve palsy. As such it is an important differential diagnosis in the neurology section of PACES.
- The examiners may ask you further questions on any topic that you raise and therefore you should be able to list the disorders associated with mononeuritis multiplex.
- The causes of connective tissue diseases are summarized in the mnemonic on page 162.
- In a third of cases of mononeuritis, no underlying cause is found.

Optic atrophy

My **S**ight's **G**one
   Multiple sclerosis
   Squashed nerve (tumour, aneurysm)
   Glaucoma

Topic facts

Optic atrophy is the common end-result of many different causes of optic nerve injury. The most common causes are listed in the mnemonic.

- Optic atrophy is seen on fundoscopy as a well-defined pale optic disc.
- Slowly progressive visual loss is a common mode of presentation.
- Examining for a relative afferent pupillary defect (RAPD) is the best discriminative test to identify early optic atrophy.
- To perform an RAPD assessment, swing a light source between the eyes, allowing time for the pupil to begin to react. In healthy eyes the pupils should remain the same size. In an affected eye the pupils will dilate because the afferent nerve is damaged and so the light source seems less intense. Once the same light source has been moved to the normal eye the direct and consensual reflex will cause the pupils to constrict.
- Look for associated findings to identify the underlying cause of the optic atrophy, e.g.:
  - MS: internuclear ophthalmoplegia, cerebellar dysarthria, past pointing, spastic weakness, etc.
  - tumour compression: visual field defects
  - glaucoma: family history, disc cupping.
- Other causes of optic atrophy: retinal artery occlusion, ischaemic optic neuropathy, Paget's disease, Friedreich's ataxia, tabes dorsalis.

Papilloedema
STAB
Space-occupying lesion
Tumour
Abscess
Bleed/**B**enign intracranial hypertension

Topic facts
Papilloedema is defined as optic disc swelling secondary to raised ICP. Common causes are listed in the mnemonic above.

- Papilloedema is typically bilateral and, unlike papillitis (optic disc neuritis), visual acuity is preserved (though visual field is reduced – typically with a central scotoma – see page 53).
- Space-occupying lesions may be primary brain tumours or secondary deposits ± cerebral oedema. Look for evidence of a primary lesion, e.g. Horner's syndrome, radiotherapy tattoo, clubbing, cachexia and nicotine staining of a bronchial primary.
- Sixth nerve palsy is a false localizing sign found in patients with raised ICP, which may be bilateral. Examine for diplopia on lateral gaze. The false image is the outermost image.
- Raised ICP is suggested by a history of early morning headaches that are eased on standing and worsened by straining or coughing.
- Abscess is suggested by presence of fever, neutrophilia and a source of infection, e.g. sinus or middle-ear infection.
- Malignant hypertension can also cause papilloedema; look for arteriovenous (AV) nipping, haemorrhages and cotton-wool spots.
- Retrobulbar neuritis is differentiated from papillitis in that the region of optic nerve affected lies behind the optic disc, so no changes can be seen on fundoscopy. Both cause impairment of visual acuity and pain on eye movement.

Paraplegia/Tetraplegia
ABC
Atlantoaxial subluxation
Bleed (into the cord)
Cord compression/trauma

Topic facts
Paraplegia is paralysis of the lower limbs and tetraplegia is paralysis
affecting all four limbs. A summary of the causes is listed here.

- LMN signs are present at the level of the lesion and UMN signs below that.
- The spinothalamic tracts that supply pain, temperature and crude touch
  decussate on entry to the spinal cord. The other tracts remain ipsilateral.
  This is reflected in the presentation of signs in cord injury.
- Cord hemisection, also known as Brown–Séquard syndrome, presents
  with ipsilateral LMN signs at the level of the lesion. Below the level of the
  lesion there are ipsilateral UMN signs and dorsal column signs but
  contralateral spinothalamic signs. Reflexes are absent at the level of the
  lesion, with hyperreflexia below the level of the lesion.
- Always ensure that you examine the back in patients with paraplegia/
  tetraplegia, otherwise you will miss the scars of previous trauma/surgery.
  Examine for a motor, sensory and reflex level.
- Cord compression at the cervical level may be caused by odontoid peg
  dislocation and subsequent atlantoaxial subluxation. The odontoid peg
  secures the upper cervical vertebrae to allow rotation. Rheumatoid
  arthritis patients are susceptible to this.
- Cord compression may be subcategorized into external compression
  (spinal stenosis, disc prolapse) and internal compression (bleeding into the
  cord).

Peripheral neuropathy
Sensory neuropathy
Damaged **C**oordination **B**ecause **D**iabetic

- **D**iabetes mellitus
- **C**arcinomatous neuropathy
- **B**$_{12}$ deficiency
- **D**rugs (amiodarone/metronidazole)

Motor neuropathy
Causes **G**reat **L**ethargy

- **C**arcinomatous neuropathy/**C**harcot–Marie–Tooth disease
- **G**uillain–Barré syndrome
- **L**ead poisoning

Topic facts
The two mnemonics listed here summarize the causes of sensory and motor neuropathy, respectively, in order of the most common occurrence.

- Peripheral neuropathy is one of the most common neurological cases so you need to know these lists and your examination routine very well to be slick.
- The key finding on examination is sensory loss in a glove-and-stocking distribution.
- Answers should be tailored to the examination findings. I cannot stress too many times the importance of careful inspection from the end of the bed. This will enable you to pick up vital clues needed to make the appropriate diagnosis, e.g. Horner's syndrome, and reduced chest expansion in a patient with bronchial neoplasm.
- In a tenth of patients with sensory neuropathy, no cause may be found.
- There are many rare causes of peripheral neuropathy.

Neurology

Proximal myopathy

DOC

Dermatomyositis/**D**rugs

Osteomalacia

Cushing's disease or syndrome/**C**arcinomatous

Topic facts

Proximal myopathy is weakness of the large proximal limb muscles. The most common causes are summarized above.

- Proximal myopathy patients complain of difficulty combing their hair, standing from sitting and climbing stairs.

- Test for proximal myopathy by asking patients to stand from sitting without using their arms to aid them. An alternative is to ask patients to stand from a squatting position.

- Dermatomyositis is a connective tissue disease associated with polymyositis. The characteristic findings are of a reddish purple 'heliotrope rash' found on the eyelids, periorbitally and on the hands. This can be subtle, so you need actively to ask yourself, every time you examine the face, 'Is it present?'. Gottron's papules are purple papules found over the metacarpophalangeal and interphalangeal joints of the hand. Nail-fold telangiectasia is probably the easiest sign to pick up – if present, look for the other signs mentioned. Dermatomyositis is associated with malignancy, which is more common in patients aged over 60.

- Drugs associated with proximal myopathy include steroids, amiodarone and alcohol (and many others).

- Osteomalacia (the adult version of rickets!) results from decreased bone mineralization caused by lack of vitamin D. Biochemical changes are of low calcium, low phosphate and high alkaline phosphate secondary to high parathyroid hormone (PTH) levels as a result of hypocalcaemia. Patients have a waddling gait.

- Cushing's disease – moon face, striae, centripetal obesity.

Ptosis

The **H**ypotonic **M**uscle **C**loses
My **T**wo **E**yes

Unilateral

Third nerve palsy
Horner's syndrome
Myasthenia gravis/**M**yotonic dystrophy
Congenital

Bilateral

Myasthenia gravis/**M**yotonic dystrophy
Tabes dorsalis
External ophthalmoplegia

Topic facts

This mnemonic lists the causes of ptosis split into unilateral and bilateral causes in order of most common occurrence.

- Ptosis is drooping of the eyelid as a result of a hypotonic levator palpebrae. This muscle is innervated by the third cranial nerve and also the sympathetic nervous system.
- Unilateral ptosis secondary to third nerve palsy is associated with a dilated pupil and a 'down-and-out' gaze on the affected side. As with all ophthalmoplegias the patient sees two images, in which the outer image is the false image. Covering the affected eye will remove the false outer image.
- Horner's syndrome is usually unilateral but can present bilaterally in patients with syringomyelia.
- Myotonic dystrophy classically presents with bilateral ptosis but weakness can be asymmetrical, leading to more marked ptosis in one eye. Look for frontal balding and a myopathic face.

Retinitis pigmentosa

LARF

Laurence–Moon–Bardet–Biedl syndrome
Alport's (EKE) syndrome
Refsum's disease
Friedreich's ataxia

Topic facts

Retinitis pigmentosa describes changes in the eye that may result from a range of diseases. A differential of retinitis pigmentosa is given here.

- The clinical finding on ophthalmoscopy of retinitis pigmentosa is black reticular pigmentation resembling bone spicules seen in the peripheries.
- Patients present with night blindness and tunnel vision. Look in the history for difficulty driving at night and bumping into objects.
- The changes of retinitis pigmentosa may also occur independently.
- This is a progressive condition.
- Patients with Laurence–Moon–Bardet–Biedl syndrome are short and obese with cognitive impairment, hypogonadism and polydactyly.
- Patients with Alport's (EKE) syndrome have **E**ye (retinitis pigmentosa), **K**idney (nephrotic syndrome, renal failure) and **E**ar (sensorineural deafness) involvement.
- Patients with Refsum's disease have sensorineural deafness, nystagmus, cerebellar ataxia and icthyosis (hyperkeratosis and scaling of the palms and soles).
- Patients with Friedreich's ataxia have characteristic skeletal deformity with cerebellar signs and mixed motor neuron signs (see page 68).

Sensory ataxia

Sensation **T**otally **C**rap

  Subacute combined degeneration/**S**pinocerebellar disease

  Tabes (dorsalis + pseudo)

  Cervical myelopathy

Topic facts

The most common causes of sensory ataxia are summarized in this mnemonic.

- Sensory ataxia results from a loss of joint position sense, which is supplied via the dorsal columns (see page 61).
- Patients have a broad-based stamping gait. When walking, patients watch their feet to help overcome loss of joint position sensation. Heel-to-toe walking exaggerates the patient's instability. Romberg's test is positive, i.e. the patient is more unsteady when standing with the eyes closed.
- Associated findings:
  - subacute combined degeneration – mixed motor signs (brisk knee reflexes and absent ankle reflexes), pallor (anaemia)

  - spinocerebellar disease, i.e. Friedreich's ataxia – cerebellar signs, skeletal changes (pes cavus, scoliosis, high arched palate)

  - tabes dorsalis (syphilis) – Argyll Robertson pupils, mixed motor signs, bilateral ptosis

  - tabes pseudo – diabetic pseudotabes (insulin pens, blood glucose stick marks on fingers, evidence of other diabetic complications)

  - cervical myelopathy – UMN signs in the legs, sensory involvement, altered reflexes in arms depending on site of lesion.

Sixth nerve palsy
MMR NMV
Mononeuritis multiplex
Multiple sclerosis
Raised ICP
Neoplasm
Myasthenia gravis
Vascular (aneurysm)

Topic facts
The causes of a sixth nerve palsy are listed here in order of the most common occurrence.

- Sixth nerve palsy cases may be present in The MRCP Part 2 or the neurology or ophthalmology parts of PACES.
- Presentation is with a history of diplopia on lateral gaze. The outer false image disappears when the affected eye is covered.
- The causes of mononeuritis multiplex are listed under its own mnemonic (see page 69).
- Associated findings:
  - MS: cerebellar signs, temporal pallor of the optic disc
  - raised ICP: morning headaches, elevated blood pressure with bradycardia, sixth nerve palsy may be bilateral
  - neoplasm: evidence of primary, proximal muscle wasting, clubbing, radiotherapy tattoos, lymphadenopathy
  - myasthenia gravis: bilateral ptosis, facial muscle weakness, snarling smile, amplitude of voice decreases on continuous speech (e.g. if asked to count to 50).

Spastic paraparesis

Major **C**ord **T**rauma **B**uggers **M**obility
  Multiple sclerosis
  Cord compression
  Trauma
  Birth injury
  MND

Topic facts

Spastic paraparesis is UMN weakness involving the lower limbs. Common causes are summarized above.

- You may be asked to assess the gait. This is characteristically described as a scissors gait or like wading through mud.
- MS is the most common cause of spastic paraparesis seen at clinical examinations. Be aware that the gait of an MS patient may be ataxic as a result of cerebellar involvement rather than spastic. A cerebellar gait is broad-based with Romberg's test negative. The patient falls towards the side of the cerebellar lesion.
- Other causes of spastic paraparesis include syringomyelia, subacute combined degeneration of the cord and Friedreich's ataxia.
- If cerebellar signs are present, MS is usually the number 1 diagnosis with Friedreich's ataxia a differential.
- Wasting of the muscles of the hand indicates involvement of the cervical cord, suggesting cervical trauma, compression, syringomyelia or MND with cervical disease.
- Syringomyelia is a fluid sac or 'syrinx' that forms in the spinal cord. Brain-stem involvement is known as syringobulbia. Dissociated sensory loss is present (spinothalamic loss in the hands, dorsal columns preserved). Look for scars/ulcers on the hands.

Stroke

TIA

Thrombus
Intracerebral bleed
Arteritis

Topic facts

The causes of a cerebrovascular accident (CVA) are given in this memory aid in order of the most common.

- Most strokes are the result of a thrombus. So, when examining a patient with features of stroke, complete your examination by looking for sources of thrombus. Feel the pulse for atrial fibrillation, identify the apex for cardiac enlargement and listen for murmurs (mitral stenosis) and bruits.
- Most strokes affect the cerebral hemispheres resulting in contralateral hemiplegia and UMN signs. You should be aware of the cerebral cortex functions and be able to attempt to localize the lesion.

Cortex functions

- Frontal lobe:
  - motor (precentral gyrus)
  - olfactory.
- Temporal lobe:
  - hearing
  - memory.
- Parietal lobe:
  - visuospatial
  - 3 Rs (Reading, wRiting, aRrithmetic).
- Occipital lobe:
  - visual cortex.

Stroke

Frontal lobe
AB PPPP
Anosmia
Broca's aphasia (see page 63)

Personality change
Primitive reflex (grasp, pout, rooting)
Perseveration
Planning difficulties
(Note that frontal lobe lesions lead to hemiplegia, typically with the leg affected much more than the arm.)

Parietal lobe
Visuospatial: neglect, astereognosis (failure to name common objects by touch), constructional apraxia (interlocking pentagons test), right/left confusion, homonymous inferior quadrantanopia.
3Rs: Reading (alexia), wRiting (agraphia), aRrithmetic (acalculia). Patients lose the ability to read, write and calculate.

Temporal lobe
Hearing, memory: memory loss, cortical deafness, Wernicke's aphasia, homonymous superior quadrantanopia.

Occipital lobe
Visual cortex: cortical blindness (bilateral occipital infarcts), homonymous hemianopia with macular sparing).

Tardive dyskinesia

He **C**onstantly **M**oves
   Haloperidol
   Chlorpromazine
   Metoclopramide

Topic facts

Tardive dyskinesias (TDs) are drug-induced involuntary movements of the face, limbs and trunk. Common drugs that cause TDs are given above.

- Stereotypical dyskinesias such as lip smacking, chewing, tongue protrusion and grimacing are characteristic of TDs.
- This movement disorder is also known as drug-induced extrapyramidal syndrome.
- Neuroleptic-induced TDs are absent during sleep.
- People receiving long-term treatment with anti-dopaminergic drugs, such as those listed in the mnemonic, are at greatest risk (e.g. people with chronic schizophrenia).
- For TDs to be diagnosed patients should have taken causative medication for a minimum of 3 months or 1 month if aged over 60.
- Other drug-induced movement disorders (or extrapyramidal syndromes) present acutely. Examples are akathisia, acute dystonia, drug-induced parkinsonism and other hyperkinetic dyskinesias.
- Dyskinesias can also occur on withdrawal of dopamine antagonists.
- Elderly patients are at increased risk of developing a dyskinesia.
- Consider other causes of choreiform movements (see page 57).
- Isolated blepharospasm (repetitive sustained contraction of orbicularis oculi) may be the one and only finding in a TD.

Third nerve palsy

Pretty **M**inimal **V**isual **M**ovement

   Posterior communicating artery aneurysm

   Mononeuritis multiplex

   Vascular lesion

   Multiple sclerosis/**M**yasthenia gravis

Topic facts

The causes of a third nerve palsy are summarized in order of the most common occurrence in this topic.

- The clinical presentation of a third nerve palsy is with ptosis, divergent strabismus and a fixed down- and out-gaze. The pupil may be dilated.
- The patient complains of diplopia with the images at an angle to each other. Covering the affected eye removes the outer false image.
- Posterior communicating artery aneurysm presents with pain of sudden onset, nausea and a third nerve palsy.
- Mononeuritis multiplex causes are discussed elsewhere (see page 69).
- MS causes third nerve palsy through demyelination in the midbrain.
- The fourth nerve causes down- and inward gaze and rotation of the eye about an axis through the pupil (intorsion). Normally fourth nerve palsies are hidden by the compensatory action of muscles supplied by the third nerve. Look for the presence of a fourth nerve palsy in patients with a third nerve palsy (absence of intorsion on down- and in-gaze).
- Third nerve palsy is often split into 'surgical' and 'non-surgical' causes, depending on pupillary involvement. This is because the pupillary fibres lie superficially and are susceptible to external compression, e.g. from an aneurysm. Ischaemic lesions that mainly affect the core are relatively pupil sparing.

Neurology

Tunnel vision

Rampant **G**laucoma **C**onstricts (vision)

Retinitis pigmentosa
Glaucoma
Choroidoretinitis

Topic facts

This topic lists the more common causes of concentric visual field loss (tunnel vision).

- Tunnel vision is the loss of peripheral visual field through 360°.
- Retinitis pigmentosa and glaucoma are the most common causes of this deficit.
- Retinitis pigmentosa is more likely to be the cause in young patients.
- Conversely glaucoma is the most common cause of tunnel vision in elderly people.
- Glaucoma is more common in those with a family history. Other risk factors include age, African–Caribbean ethnicity and elevated intraocular pressure (note that patients can develop glaucoma with normal intraocular pressure).
- Most glaucoma sufferers are asymptomatic and unaware of deterioration in their visual field until late in the disease course.
- The key finding on fundoscopy is cupping of the optic disc. The cup is the central white part of the disc, which is compared with the total disc size. As glaucoma progresses the area of the cup increases.
- Choroiditis is thought to result from infection with *Toxoplasma* and cytomegalovirus; however, often the underlying cause is unknown.
- Fundoscopy will help differentiate retinitis pigmentosa from choroidoretinitis.
- Retinitis pigmentosa and the associated diseases are discussed on page 76.

Wasting of the small muscles of the hand
Must **S**tart **C**entral **P**roceed **T**o **C**ervical + **P**lexus

Anterior horn cells (C8, T1)
MND
Syringomyelia
Charcot–Marie–Tooth disease
Polio

Root lesion
Tumour (neurofibroma)
Cervical spondylosis

Plexus damage (brachial)
Pancoast's tumour/**P**ressure from a cervical rib

Topic facts
The causes of wasting of the small muscles of the hand are listed here from the origin of the LMN in the anterior horn cells, downwards through the nerve root and brachial plexus.

- Small muscle wasting of the hands may also be caused by disuse atrophy, especially in patients with arthritis.
- The LMNs supplying the small muscles of the hand originate at level C8 and T1.
- Look for the associated features:

  - MND: fasciculation, bulbar palsy, mixed motor signs from the cord

  - syringomyelia: dissociated sensory loss, scars on hands

  - Pancoast's tumour: Horner's syndrome.

Neurology

Gastroenterology

- Abdominal pain + neuropathy
- Abdominal pain + renal failure
- Ascites
- Bloody diarrhoea
- Cholestasis + normal ultrasonography
- Cholestatic jaundice
- Chronic liver disease
- Coeliac disease
- Crohn's disease
- Diverticular disease
- Food poisoning
- Gastrointestinal bleeding
- Hepatic encephalopathy
- Hepatomegaly
- Hepatosplenomegaly
- Hyposplenism
- Jaundice – prehepatic causes
- Malabsorption
- Obstruction
- Pancreatitis
- Parotid swelling
- Primary biliary cirrhosis
- Retroperitoneal fibrosis
- Splenomegaly
- Travellers' diarrhoea
- Ulcerative colitis
- Vitamin B_{12} + folate deficiency

Abdominal pain + neuropathy

Diabetics **G**et **A**bdominal **P**ain + **N**europathy

Diabetic patients
Guillain–Barré syndrome
Acute intermittent porphyria
PAN (polyarteritis nodosa), **P**oisoning (lead)
Alcohol
Neoplasm

Topic facts

Causes of combined abdominal pain and neuropathy are summarized in this differential.

- Diabetes is the most common cause of peripheral neuropathy in the UK. A combination of peripheral neuropathy and acute abdominal pain is found in patients with established type 1 diabetes and ketoacidosis.
- Guillain–Barré syndrome (GBS) is an acute, ascending, predominantly motor, demyelinating polyneuropathy. Abdominal and back pain are common early features of GBS.
  - GBS is associated with recent infection with *Campylobacter jejuni* or *Chlamydia* spp.
  - Proximal muscles are most affected and the cranial nerves may be involved. Bulbar palsy may develop, and there may be autonomic nervous system involvement leading to tachyarrhythmias, constipation and abdominal pain.
- Lead poisoning interferes with haem synthesis. High levels of haem precursors lead to abdominal symptoms, and autonomic and motor neuropathy similar to that of acute intermittent porphyria (AIP). (See page 58.)
- Aminolaevulanic acid (ALA) is raised in both AIP and lead poisoning but in lead poisoning there is elevated proto- and co-proporphyrins and anaemia with basophilic stippling.
- Blue lines on the gums occur in lead poisoning and lead lines may be seen in the long bones.

Gastroenterology

Abdominal pain + renal failure

Abdominal **P**ain + **R**enal **M**alfunction

Adult polycystic kidney disease
PAN and other vasculitides
Raised calcium
Methanol

Topic facts

Causes of combined abdominal pain and failure of renal function are given here.

- Adult polycystic kidney disease (APCKD) is an autosomal dominant inherited condition (chromosome 16) in which multiple cysts form in the kidneys and other organs. Patients may present with flank pain and haematuria as the result of haemorrhage into a cyst.
- APCKD is one of the few disorders in which there is renal failure without anaemia as a result of inappropriate erythropoietin production.
- APCKD is associated with mitral valve prolapse, berry aneurysms and subarachnoid haemorrhage.
- Diagnosis can be made on ultrasonographic criteria that are age dependent (as the number of cysts increases with age).
- PAN is a small-vessel vasculitis that can affect any organ system. Avoid confusion with microscopic polyangitis (MPA). Presentation is with weight loss, livedo reticularis, myalgia, neuropathy and organ-specific symptoms depending on their involvement. Renal failure may occur if the renal system is involved. Other vasculitides involving the kidney are Wegener's granulomatosis and Churg–Strauss syndrome.
- Hypercalcaemia is a medical emergency and presents with nausea, constipation, abdominal pain, polyuria and headache. Management is with rehydration followed by bisphosphonate therapy.
- Also consider haemolytic uraemic syndrome (HUS).
- Methanol is a soluent found in antifreeze and windscreen wash. Symptoms of methanol poisoning occur 8-36 hours after ingestion. Methanol is broken down to the toxic substance formic acid which can cause metabolic acidosis and subsequent renal failure.

Ascites

6 Cs

Cirrhosis
Congestive cardiac failure
Cancer
Caval compression
C(k)idneys (nephritic syndrome)
Constrictive pericarditis

Topic facts

Ascites is the collection of fluid in the peritoneal space. The causes are summarized in this mnemonic.

- Cirrhosis caused by alcohol abuse is the most common cause of ascites. Look for evidence of chronic liver disease (palmar erythema, liver flap, spider naevi, parotid enlargement, icterus, dilated abdominal veins).
- Congestive cardiac failure is suggested by finding a pulsatile liver, displaced apex and peripheral oedema.
- Other causes of ascites include portal vein thrombosis, granulomatous liver disease and Budd–Chiari syndrome.
- Serum ascites albumin gradient (SAAG) is a measure of portal hypertension. It has replaced the traditional transudate/exudate assessment of ascitic fluid.
- A SAAG >11 suggests ascites caused by portal hypertension (transudative). Simply measure albumin concentration in the serum and ascitic fluid and calculate the difference.
- Patients with ascites are at risk of spontaneous bacterial peritonitis (SBP). Patients who become unwell with coexistent ascites should have a sample of the ascitic fluid taken for cell count and culture. If the neutrophil count is >250 cells/L, the diagnosis of SBP should be made and the patient requires aggressive treatment with antibiotics.

Bloody diarrhoea

CAM – SHIG – ENT
CAM pylobacter
SHIG ella
ENT amoeba histolytica

Topic facts

The common causes of infective bloody diarrhoea are given here.

- *Campylobacter* spp., *Shigella* spp. and *Entamoeba histolytica* are among the most common causes of haemorrhagic infective diarrhoea.
- Other infective causes of bloody diarrhoea include *Salmonella* spp., *Clostridium difficile* with pseudomembranous colitis, *Strongyloides* spp. and *Escherichia coli*.
- *Entamoeba* sp. is the exception in the infective diarrhoea group because, unlike the others, it does not respond well to ciprofloxacin. Entamoeba infection should be treated with metronidazole.
- Non-infective causes of bloody diarrhoea include:
  - inflammatory bowel disease (IBD)
  - colorectal cancer
  - ischaemic colitis
  - HUS (associated with *E. coli* infection, particularly type 0157)
- Organisms that cause food poisoning are discussed on page 97.
- Campylobacter and salmonella infection may be acquired from ingestion of infected food, particularly eggs, dairy and chicken meat.
- Campylobacter infections are most common in the summer season.
- *Entamoeba histolytica* is a parasite (and has resistance to water chlorination), which is prevalent in much of Asia, Africa and South America.

Cholestasis + normal ultrasonography

Cholestasis With Perfect Abdomen

Chronic active hepatitis

Wilson's disease

Primary sclerosing cholangitis, primary biliary cirrhosis (PBC)

Alpha$_1$ antitrypsin deficiency

Topic facts

This topic covers the differential for patients with cholestasis and normal ultrasonography.

- Chronic active hepatitis (CAH) is an autoimmune disease resulting in chronic hepatic inflammation. It typically affects women aged 45–70.
- Patients have a history of lethargy, weight loss and prolonged bleeding. Histology reveals piecemeal necrosis.
- Smooth muscle antibodies (SMAs) are present in >90 per cent of type 1 CAH.
- Liver–kidney–muscle 1 (LKM-1) antibodies are found in about half of those with type 2 CAH.
- Immunoglobulins are elevated in both types 1 and 2 CAH, typically IgG.

- Wilson's disease is an autosomal recessive inherited disorder (chromosome 13) of copper metabolism. Symptoms result from high levels of copper deposition in the organs, including the liver, brain and eye. Kayser–Fleischer rings may be seen on fundoscopy.

- Patients may present with liver disease or neurological features (tremor, ataxia, personality changes). Test for serum ceruloplasmin or urinary copper excretion. Typically presents in females in their late teens.

- Primary sclerosing cholangitis is associated with IBD. The cause is unknown. A typical beaded appearance of the bile ducts is seen on cholangiography.

- PBC – see page 108.

Cholestatic jaundice

Drugs **C**an **P**romote **H**epatic **O**bstruction

Intrahepatic

Drugs
Cirrhosis
Pregnancy
Hepatitis

Extrahepatic

Obstruction:
- Common bile stone
- Cancer of the head of the pancreas
- Iatrogenic biliary stricture after surgery
- Pancreatitis
- Sclerosing cholangitis

Topic facts

The causes of cholestatic jaundice are manifold. They can be broadly split into intrahepatic and extrahepatic categories. This topic lists the more common causes.

- Drug-induced causes of cholestasis include the oral contraceptive pill, erythromycin, tricyclic antidepressants, chlorpromazine and sulfonylureas.
- Acute hepatitis can be categorized into: viral (hepatitis A), drug-induced hepatitis (isoniazid, valproate, phenytoin, amiodarone), alcohol, poisoning (paracetamol overdose) and bacterial (Weil's disease, *Mycoplasma* sp.).
- In the PACES it is best to offer a broad overview of causes; the examiner will then choose to lead you down the relevant path, e.g. causes of chronic liver disease and cirrhosis.

Chronic liver disease
Cirrhosis Has Always Been Connected With Alcohol
    Chronic active hepatitis
    Haemochromatosis/Hepatitis B, C
    Alpha$_1$ antitrypsin deficiency (α_1AT)
    Budd–Chiari syndrome/Biliary Cirrhosis
    Wilson's disease
    Alcohol

Topic facts
The common causes of chronic liver disease are summarized here.
- Alcohol is the most common cause of cirrhosis in the UK, with viral hepatitis (hepatitis C) being the second. Worldwide, hepatitis B infection is the most common cause of liver cirrhosis.
- Hepatitis B and C are both spread via blood and sexual contact; 5 per cent of hepatitis B infections become chronic versus >60 per cent of hepatitis C infections.
- Improved treatment of acute infection with hepatitis C has led to higher clearance rates (pegylated interferon).
- Hepatitis B is the only DNA virus of the viral hepatitis group.
- Haemochromatosis is an autosomal recessive (chromosome 6) disorder of iron metabolism. A ferritin >500 µg/L is strongly suspicious. Genetic testing is now routine for the common mutations – C282Y, H63D. Iron deposition in the liver leads to cirrhosis. Diabetes can develop from pancreatic involvement, as can hypopituitarism and hypogonadism.
- α_1AT is an enzyme deficiency that inactivates proteases. It causes chronic obstructive pulmonary disease (COPD) and cirrhosis. Obstructive lung disease in a young adult suggests this cause.
- Budd–Chiari syndrome is hepatic vein thrombosis. It is associated with prothrombotic states (myeloproliferative disease, polycythaemia rubra vera [PRV], paroxysmal nocturnal haemoglobinuria [PNH], tumours).

Gastroenterology

Coeliac disease

Coeliac **D**isease **H**as **P**lenty **O**f **A**ssociated **F**eatures **E**specially **W**eight **L**oss

Clubbing

Dermatitis herpetiformis

Haemorrhage (vitamin K deficiency)

Paraesthaesia (Ca^{2+} and Mg^{2+} deficiency)

Oedema (protein deficiency)

Anaemia (iron and folate deficiency)

Flatulence (impaired disaccharide hydrolysis)

Electrolyte disturbances (weakness and hypotension)

Weight loss (protein and fat deficiency)

Topic facts

This topic lists the clinical and biochemical findings in patients with coeliac disease.

- Coeliac disease is the most common malabsorption disorder in the UK and frequently appears in the MRCP. The underlying cause is hypersensitivity to gliadin. It can present at any age.
- Symptoms of diarrhoea are present in most patients. Weight loss, fatigue and oedema are also common.
- It is important to differentiate coeliac disease from Crohn's disease in the exam, as this may also present with chronic diarrhoea. Crohn's disease typically causes painful diarrhoea as a result of strictures causing obstructive-type symptoms. Patients with coeliac disease may complain of bloating and wind but pain is not a prominent feature.
- Diagnosis is made by endoscopy and jejunal biopsy. The histological finding is of partial or total villous atrophy (which resolves on removing gluten from the diet).
- Anti-endomysial, anti-gliadin and tissue transglutaminase antibodies are found in coeliac disease.

Crohn's disease

Oh **M**y **P**ainful **A**rse **F**issure

    Obstruction

    Malabsorption

    Proctocolitis/**P**erforation

    Abscess

    Fistulas/**F**issures

Topic facts

Crohn's disease is one of the inflammatory bowel diseases. The complications associated with Crohn's disease are summarized above.

- Features common to all inflammatory bowel diseases are found on page 112.
- Patients present with a history of abdominal pain (as the result of gut obstruction caused by strictures) and bloody stools. Perianal tags may be present.
- Failure to thrive may occur if patients are affected at a young age (leading to short, thin patients).
- Scars may be present on the abdomen as the result of previous surgery for obstruction.
- Crohn's disease can affect any part of the gut but has a predilection for the ileum, colon and rectum.
- Involvement of the terminal ileum can lead to vitamin B_{12} deficiency as a result of malabsorption.
- Skip lesions are present, i.e. gut involvement is not continuous (unlike ulcerative colitis).
- There is transmural involvement (full thickness) of the affected gut (in ulcerative colitis only the mucosa and submucosa are affected).
- Crypt abscesses are typical of ulcerative colitis, not Crohn's disease.
- Smoking and the use of oral contraceptives are associated with an increased risk of Crohn's disease.
- Investigation of Crohn's disease is with inflammatory markers, barium, studies, endoscopy and biopsy.

Gastroenterology

Diverticular disease
LAV POO

Clinical features
Left iliac fossa pain
Altered bowel habit
Vomiting

Complications
Perforation
Obstruction
Other (fistula, abscess, bleed)

Topic facts
The clinical features and complications of diverticular disease are
summarized in this topic.

- Diverticula are mucosal outpouchings in the gut wall that form in areas
  of weakness. They are common and found in most of the population
  over the age of 50.
- The sigmoid colon is the most commonly affected site.
- Ninety per cent of patients are symptom-free.
- Acute diverticulitis develops when faecal material becomes impacted in
  the diverticulum and infection and inflammation result. Bleeding may
  occur as a result of rupture of the small blood vessels around the site of
  the diverticulum.
- Imaging with computed tomography (CT) of the abdomen is the
  investigation of choice for acute diverticulitis. If perforation is
  suspected, request an erect chest radiograph for free gas under the
  diaphragm.
- Management is usually conservative with intravenous antibiotics.
- Complications result from abscess formation, perforation, fistula and
  obstruction.

Food poisoning
Stay **Bac**k **Sal**ly **Clos**e **Camp**

> **Sta***phylococcus aureus*
> **Bac***illus cereus*
> **Sal***monella enteriditis*
> **Clos***tridium perfringens/botulinum*
> **Camp***ylobacter*

Topic facts
The common causes of food poisoning are listed here in order of speed of onset of symptoms.

- *Staphylococcus aureus* and *Bacillus cereus* lead to symptoms within 6 hours of ingestion as a result of the presence of preformed toxins.
- Onset of salmonella and clostridium infection is on the same day as ingestion.
- Campylobacter infection leads to symptoms within 2–3 days.
- All forms lead to diarrhoea. Vomiting is associated with the first three causes.
- *Clostridium perfringens* diarrhoea is typically very watery.
- *Clostridium botulinum* leads to features of paralysis as a result of neuromuscular blockade by botulinum toxin.
- Investigation should be with stool culture.
- If *C. botulinum* is suspected test for botulinum toxin.
- *S. aureus* and *B. cereus* may be identified in the contaminated food source.
- *E. coli* infection is an important omission to this list. Its onset is 1–2 days after ingestion (toxins produced in the small intestine) and it is associated with HUS. Diarrhoea may be haemorrhagic if severe.
- *Giardia lamblia* should be suspected in those with a history of foreign travel and symptoms of flatulence and bloating.

Gastrointestinal bleeding
Upper gastrointestinal (GI) bleeds
Upper **G**I **O**esophageal **V**arices
> **U**lcers (gastric/duodenal)
> **G**astritis (aspirin, non-steroidal anti-inflammatory drugs [NSAIDs])
> **O**esophagitis (erosive ± hiatus hernia)
> **V**arices

Lower GI bleeds
He **F**ound **PR** **B**leeding
> **H**aemorrhoids
> **F**issures (anal)
> **P**olyps
> **B**owel diseases (inflammatory, diverticular)

Topic facts
The common causes of GI bleeding are categorized by location and summarized by these two mnemonics.
- Upper GI bleeding is most commonly the result of ulceration.
- *H. pylori* infection is the most common cause of duodenal ulceration. Eradication aids healing and reduces risk of recurrence. Triple therapy is used: two antibiotics and a proton pump inhibitor.
- Erosive gastric ulcers resulting from the use of NSAIDs are the second most common type of upper GI bleed. Cyclo-oxygenase 1 (COX-1) inhibition by NSAIDs causes reduced mucosal protection from gastric acid.
- Gastric ulcers are at risk of malignant change.
- Varices are found in patients with portal hypertension. Intervention includes use of sclerosants, banding and vasopressin-like drugs.
- A good history is important in lower GI bleed investigation.

Hepatic encephalopathy
BAD Infection
Bleed (GI bleed)
Azotaemia
Drugs (sedatives, diuretics)/**D**iet (protein load)
Infection

Topic facts

Precipitants of hepatic encephalopathy in patients with chronic liver disease are listed above.

- Hepatic encephalopathy is a feature of decompensated liver disease. Those with borderline liver function, if compromised by insults such as those listed above, may develop a reversible encephalopathy.
- Azotaemia is the accumulation of nitrogen-containing waste products in the blood, which are usually excreted in the urine.
- Hepatic encephalopathy is graded into four parts.

Score	Clinical findings
1	Flap
2	Confusion
3	Drowsy but rousable
4	Coma

- You should be aware of the Child–Pugh score for chronic liver disease. Prognosis is predicted on the basis of five factors that can be labelled A–E. The important prognosticators are:
  A – albumin
  B – bilirubin
  C – clotting (INR – international normalized ratio)
  D – distension (due to ascites)
  E – encephalopathy.

Hepatomegaly

Top 3 CCC

Cirrhosis (normally alcohol-related)
Cancer (metastasis)
Congestive cardiac failure

Topic facts

The top three causes of isolated hepatomegaly in the UK are listed here.

- In the clinical case, the associated findings listed below will help you tailor your differential:
  - <u>alcohol</u>: flap, palmar erythema, spider naevi, parotid enlargement, ascites
  - <u>carcinoma</u>: lymphadenopathy, cachexia, hard, knobbly liver edge, radiotherapy tattoo
  - <u>congestive cardiac failure</u>: peripheral oedema, raised jugular venous pressure (JVP), displaced cardiac apex, pulsatile liver, cardiac medication – GTN (glyceryl trinitrate) spray
  - <u>lymphoproliferative disease</u>: lymphadenopathy, splenomegaly
  - <u>viral hepatitis</u>: hepatitis A, B, infectious mononucleosis, mycoplasma, leptospirosis; look for tender hepatomegaly with a history of fever
  - <u>amyloidosis</u>: primary/secondary (chronic disease).

Hepatosplenomegaly

CML Get **H**epatosplenomegaly

Chronic myeloid leukaemia (CML)

Myelofibrosis

Lymphatic leukaemia (chronic lymphatic leukaemia or CLL)

Gaucher's disease

Hairy cell leukaemia

Plus

Myeloproliferative disease

RBCs (red blood cells): polycythaemia rubra vera

WBCs (white blood cells): acute myeloid leukaemia (neutrophils are
   myeloid in origin)

Platelets: essential thrombocythaemia

Fibroblasts: primary myelofibrosis.

Topic facts

The top five causes of hepatosplenomegaly in the UK are summarized here.
The first three are in order of most common occurrence. These are the
same causes as for splenomegaly, plus the myeloproliferative diseases.

- CML is discussed on page 11. The hepatosplenomegaly in this case
  results from bone marrow infiltration and the need for haemopoiesis
  outside the marrow. A similar mechanism is true for the other five
  causes.
- Gaucher's disease is an autosomal recessive metabolic disorder in which
  lipids accumulate in the bone marrow, liver and spleen as a result of a
  deficiency of the enzyme glucocerebrosidase.
- Patients present with hepatosplenomegaly, anaemia and
  thrombocytopenia.
- Note that cirrhosis with portal hypertension should be considered in the
  context of chronic liver disease.

Gastroenterology

Hyposplenism

Causes

Underactive Spleen Causes Trouble

- Ulcerative colitis
- Sickle cell disease
- Coeliac disease
- Thrombocythaemia/Tropical sprue

Infection risk

Hyposplenics Need Prophylactic Meds

- Haemophilus influenzae
- Neisseria meningitides
- Pneumococci
- Malaria

Topic facts

The first mnemonic lists the common causes of hyposplenism. The second lists the conditions to which hyposplenic patients are susceptible.

- Hyposplenism predisposes to risk of infection from the encapsulated bacteria and for those travelling outside the UK to affected regions – malaria.
- Prophylactic treatment is advised.
- Patients should be offered meningococcal, pneumoccocal and influenza vaccines.
- Bacterial prophylaxis is with oral phenoxymethylpenicillin daily.
- Most adults with sickle cell disease are hyposplenic. Recurrent splenic infarction is the result of sickling and subsequent vaso-occlusion.
- Splenectomy patients are obviously also at risk. Indications for splenectomy include traumatic rupture, autoimmune/congenital haemolytic disease, myelofibrosis and lymphoproliferative disease.
- Howell–Jolly bodies are found on the blood film after splenectomy.

Jaundice – prehepatic causes

Haemolysis **R**eleases **I**ntracellular **B**ilirubin

Haemolysis
Rhesus incompatibility (and other immune haemolytic reactions)
Infection
Burns

Topic facts

This topic covers the prehepatic causes of jaundice.

- Jaundice is the result of elevated levels of bilirubin in the blood. Hyperbilirubinaemia is the consequence of an excessive bilirubin load, intrahepatic disease or extrahepatic biliary duct obstruction.
- Intrahepatic and extrahepatic causes of jaundice are discussed on page 92.
- Prehepatic hyperbilirubinaemia is unconjugated, because conjugation occurs in the liver (to increase solubility and allow absorption into the biliary ducts). Testing for this helps identify the underlying cause.
- Unconjugated bilirubin is not found in urine because it is water-insoluble. It is transported in the blood by binding to plasma proteins.
- Haemolytic hyperbilirubinaemia is associated with macrocytic anaemia and elevated reticulocyte count. Causes of congenital haemolytic anaemia are discussed on page 3.
- Coombs' test is for antibodies on the patient's RBCs. If positive it indicates an autoimmune cause for the haemolytic anaemia.
- Other causes of haemolysis include microangiopathic haemolytic anaemia (see page 12), PNH, and cold and warm autoimmune haemolytic anaemias.
- Haemolytic transfusion reactions occur immediately and are life-threatening. Febrile reactions to transfusion are non-haemolytic.

Malabsorption
CROHN'S

Coeliac/**C**rohn's disease
Radiation enteritis/**R**esection (intestinal/Whipple's disease)
Overgrowth (bacterial)
Herpetiformis (dermatitis)
Neoplasm (lymphoma)
Sprue (tropical + parasites)

Topic facts

The more common causes of small bowel malabsorption are listed here.

- Coeliac disease and Crohn's disease are by far the most common causes of small bowel malabsorption.
- Patients present with diarrhoea, weight loss, lethargy and nutritional deficiency.
- Terminal ileum involvement predisposes to vitamin B_{12} deficiency. Macrocytic anaemia results.
- Investigate for vitamin B_{12} deficiency with the Schilling test. A large dose of vitamin B_{12} is given to saturate the body's ability to bind vitamin B_{12}. Then radiolabelled vitamin B_{12} is given. In a normal person this is absorbed in the terminal ileum and excreted in the urine. More than 10 per cent excretion is considered normal.
- Patients with impaired small bowel transit times and anatomical abnormalities are predisposed to bacterial overgrowth.
- Causes of slowed gut transit times include diabetic neuropathy, systemic sclerosis and intestinal obstruction.
- Anatomical causes of overgrowth include diverticula, intestinal resections, blind loops and fistulas.
- Dermatitis herpetiformis is an intensely pruritic blistering disorder associated with coeliac disease and malabsorption. Treat with dapsone and avoid gluten.
- Look for a history of radiation, surgery and foreign travel to suggest the cause of the malabsorption.

Obstruction

I Must **H**ave **A V**oluminous **P**oo

    Inflammation/**I**ntussception

    Malignancy/**M**eckel's diverticulum/**M**econium

    Hernia/**H**irschsprung's disease

    Atresia/**A**dhesions/**A**ppendicitis

    Volvulus (sigmoid/neonatorum)

    Pyloric stenosis

Topic facts

This memory aid lists the causes of GI obstruction.

- Although obstruction is not a common case in the MRCP exam it may present as a complication of other disease processes, i.e. malignancy, IBD.

- Medical patients may go on to develop obstruction and it is not uncommon to see a patient in the medical admissions unit with abdominal pain that turns out to be obstruction missed in the accident and emergency department.

- It is included here because it is easy to recall and provides a useful differential list at your fingertips (whether in MRCP exam or the medical admissions unit).

Gastroenterology

Pancreatitis
DAMAGE
Drugs (steroids, azathioprine, thiazides)
Alcohol
Mumps
Autoimmune (diabetes mellitus)
Gallstones
Endoscopic retrograde cholangiopancreatography (ERCP)

Topic facts
The more common causes of acute pancreatitis are summarized in this topic.
- Gallstones are the most common cause of acute pancreatitis followed by alcohol-induced pancreatitis.
- Markers of prognosis in acute pancreatitis include age (>55 years), white cell count (WCC) >15 × 10^9/L, urea <16 mmol/L, hypoxia (P_{O_2} <8 kPa), calcium <2 mmol/L and glucose >10 mmol/L.
- Hypercalcaemia is a cause of pancreatitis, but pancreatitis causes hypocalcaemia.
- Acute pancreatitis presents clinically with epigastric pain radiating to the back and vomiting. There may be epigastric tenderness and guarding.
- Investigation – the diagnosis remains largely clinical, but is supported by an elevated serum amylase (more than five times the upper limit of normal).
- Management includes intravenous fluid replacement and nasogastric tube placement.
- Complications include renal failure, pancreatic pseudocysts and pancreatic abscess.
- Chronic pancreatitis is most commonly the result of alcohol abuse.
- Patients may present with exacerbations caused by excess alcohol intake.
- Treatment involves cessation of alcohol, replacement of pancreatic enzymes for those with malabsorption (creon) and hypoglycaemics (usually insulin is required) for those who develop diabetes.

Parotid swelling

Alcoholics **M**ay **H**ave **S**wollen **C**heeks

Alcholic liver disease
Metabolic (diabetes mellitus)
HIV infection (and other viruses)
Sarcoidosis/**S**jögren's syndrome
Cancer (lymphoma)

Topic facts

The common causes of parotid swelling are summarized here.

- Sarcoidosis is a multisystem granulomatous disorder. The lung is commonly affected but involvement of other organs is common. Infiltration of the parotids leads to bilateral swelling.
- Anterior uveitis is a common finding in sarcoidosis. Look for this in combination with parotid swelling.
- Presenting features include dry cough, shortness of breath, lymphadenopathy and eye involvement.
- Sjögren's syndrome is a disorder of exocrine gland function. It is more common in older women. Patients complain of dry eyes and dry mouth.
- Sjögren's syndrome can be primary (a connective tissue disease – see page 162) or secondary.
- Secondary Sjögren's syndrome is linked to other connective tissue disorders such as systemic lupus erythematosus (SLE) and rheumatoid arthritis.
- Investigations for Sjögren's syndrome include anti-nuclear antibodies (ANAs), anti-Ro and anti-La antibodies. ANAs are non-specific but present in the majority. Ro and La are present in about half of cases.
- Other viruses associated with parotid swelling:
  - mumps virus
  - parainfluenza virus type 3
  - Coxsackie virus
  - influenza A virus.

Primary biliary cirrhosis
SCRATCH

Sjögren's syndrome (70 per cent)
Coeliac disease
Renal tubular acidosis
Anti-mitochondrial antibodies
Thyroid (20 per cent hypothyroidism)
CREST*
Hypertension (portal)

Topic facts

Primary biliary cirrhosis (PBC) is an organ-specific autoimmune disease (see page 124). The associated conditions and findings are given in the mnemonic.

- PBC patients often SCRATCH, as the most common presentation is of pruritis and lethargy.
- Patients present in their 40 s.
- Ninety per cent of patients with PBC are female and symptoms precede the onset of jaundice.
- A cholestatic picture of liver dysfunction then develops with pale stools and dark urine.
- PBC belongs to a group of disorders called the organ-specific autoimmune disease. Patients with one organ-specific autoimmune disease are at increased risk of developing another.
- Seventy per cent of those with PBC develop Sjögren's syndrome and 20 per cent have thyroid dysfunction.
- The key investigation is positive anti-mitochondrial antibodies (subtype M2) on blood tests.
- Diagnosis can be confirmed by liver biopsy.
- Patients are managed with ursodeoxycholic acid and immunosuppressants.
- Cholestyramine and antihistamines are used as anti-pruritic agents.

*****C**REST (**c**alcinosis, **R**aynaud's phenomenon, oe**s**ophagitis, **s**clerosis, **t**elangiectasia).

Retroperitoneal fibrosis

ALARM

Aortic aneurysm
Lymphoma
Aetiology unknown
Retroperitoneal tumour
Methysergide (anti-migraine drug)

Topic facts

Retroperitoneal fibrosis describes the formation of fibrous tissue in the retroperitoneal space, which may encase the aorta, ureters and vena cava. Causes are listed in the mnemonic.

- Retroperitoneal fibrosis is a relatively rare condition.
- Patients present with abdominal pain most commonly in the flanks. Weight loss, nausea and urinary symptoms are common.
- Complications of the fibrosis include ureteric obstruction ± renal failure, venous and lymphatic obstruction.
- In most cases no cause is found. In these patients an autoimmune process is thought to be the cause, and a course of steroid treatment may help.
- Investigation is with computerised tomography (CT) or magnetic resonance imaging (MRI).

Splenomegaly

CML Get **H**epatosplenomegaly

    Chronic myeloid leukaemia

    Myelofibrosis

    Lymphatic leukaemia (CLL)

    Gaucher's disease

    Hairy cell leukaemia

Topic facts

This mnemonic lists the top five causes of splenomegaly in the UK. The first three are in order of most common occurrence. The causes are the same as for hepatosplenomegaly.

- Worldwide, malaria is the most common cause, followed by leishmaniasis.
- Consider cirrhosis with portal hypertension, particularly if there are signs of chronic liver disease on examination.
- Hepatosplenomegaly with lymphadenopathy points towards lymphatic leukaemia or lymphoma.
- Hairy cell leukaemia refers to the appearance of the cells under the microscope, due to hair-like outgrowths seen on the cell periphery.
- Other causes of splenomegaly to be considered include infectious causes:
  - <u>bacterial</u>: brucellosis, TB and typhoid
  - <u>viral</u>: Epstein–Barr virus
  - <u>parasitic</u>: malaria, leishmaniasis.

Travellers' diarrhoea
CAM–SHIG–ENT
Runny **S**tools **N**ot **G**ood
> **C**ampylobacter sp.
> **S**higella sp.
> **E**ntamoeba histolytica
> **R**otavirus
> **S**almonella sp.
> **N**orwalk virus
> **G**iardia lamblia

Topic facts
Travellers' diarrhoea refers to infectious causes of diarrhoea encountered in patients with a recent history of foreign travel.

- Infectious diarrhoea is suggested by a diarrhoea of acute onset, often affecting several members of a group.
- Stool culture is the most appropriate investigation.
- Treatment is conservative with replacement of fluids orally or intravenously if required. If prolonged, most bacterial gastrointestinal infections are ciprofloxacin sensitive.
- The first three organisms are also causes of bloody diarrhoea (see page 90).
- Other causes of diarrhoea can be subdivided into disorders of secretion, and osmotic and motility disorders.
- Secretory diarrhoeas continue despite fasting and include infection with *E. coli* and cholera.
- Osmotic diarrhoeas cease with fasting and are caused by osmotically active bowel substances, i.e. magnesium sulphate and osmotic laxatives such as lactulose.
- Motility diarrhoeas may be caused by thyrotoxicosis, irritable bowel syndrome or diabetic autonomic neuropathy.

Ulcerative colitis

UC
Upwards spread
Colon only

PACE
Pyoderma gangrenosum
Arthritis (about 2 per cent)
Clubbing
Erythema nodosum/**E**ye involvement

Topic facts
The first mnemonic describes the pattern of gut involvement in UC.
Ulcerative colitis starts in the rectum and spread is continuous from the
rectum upwards. Involvement is confined to the colon. The second
mnemonic lists the findings common to the inflammatory bowel diseases
(IBD).

- Ulcerative colitis is a chronic IBD.
- There are two peak ages of presentation – early adulthood and
  late 50s.
- It is more common in females.
- Weight loss, abdominal pain and bloody diarrhoea are common
  presenting symptoms.
- Primary sclerosing cholangitis (PSC) is associated with UC (most patients
  with PSC have coexistent UC).
- There are two types of arthritis associated with the inflammatory bowel
  diseases: an ankylosing spondylitis type (axial arthropathy) with an HLA-
  B27 association and a peripheral arthropathy affecting large joints.
- Eye involvement in IBD refers to iritis and uveitis.

Vitamin B$_{12}$ and folate deficiency

Bacteria **B**reakdown **B**$_{12}$ **B**ut **F**art out **F**olate

Topic facts

The effect of bacteria on dietary vitamin B$_{12}$ and folate is summarized in this memory aid.

- Bacteria in the gut break down vitamin B$_{12}$ but do not metabolize folate. Thus, in bacterial overgrowth of the gut there is a vitamin B$_{12}$ deficiency but folate levels are normal or high.
- Bacterial overgrowth occurs in those who have had small bowel resections and those with small bowel diverticula. The bacteria can feast on the unabsorbed food, leading to bacterial overgrowth.
- Patients may present with diarrhoea and features of malabsorption.
- Treatment is eradication with antibiotics, typically metronidazole or ciprofloxacin.
- Meat is the main source of vitamin B$_{12}$ in the diet. The main source of folate is vegetables.
- Pernicious anaemia accounts for three-quarters of all cases of vitamin B$_{12}$ deficiency and is a result of a lack of intrinsic factor. Intrinsic factor binds to vitamin B$_{12}$ in the stomach without which vitamin B$_{12}$ cannot be absorbed.
- Pernicious anaemia is associated with a macrocytic anaemia and a yellowish skin tinge.
- *Helicobacter pylori* can cause pernicious anaemia through damage to the gastric mucosa.
- Vitamin B$_{12}$ is absorbed in the terminal ileum. Damage to this area can lead to deficiency, i.e. due to resection, coeliac disease, Crohn's disease, ileal tuberculosis (TB), sprue.

Endocrinology

- Amenorrhoea
- Congenital adrenal hyperplasia
- DiGeorge syndrome
- Diabetes insipidus
- Diabetes-related skin disease
- Hyperaldosteronism
- Hyperthyroidism
- Hypogonadism
- McCune–Albright syndrome
- Organ-specific autoimmune disease
- Osteomalacia
- Phaeochromocytoma
- Polydipsia
- Prolactin elevation
- Schmidt's syndrome
- Stress hormones
- Thyroid cancer

Amenorrhoea
PMT
Pregnancy
Polycystic ovary syndrome
Pituitary problems (prolactinomas)
Malabsorption
Malnutrition
Manly
Testicular feminization
Turner syndrome

Topic facts

Amenorrhoea is the failure of menstruation. The differential of amenorrhoea is given here.

- Polycystic ovarian syndrome (PCOS) is a common disorder of sex hormones in which there are typical phenotypic findings: hairy, fat, spotty, with scanty or absent periods.
- Investigate with: **LH** or luteinizing hormone (level **h**igh), FSH or follicle-stimulating hormone (level is normal or low) and androgens (somewines raised). The LH:FSH ratio is raised at > 2:1.
- The term 'manly' refers to a woman who has been virilized. A DHEA (dihydroepiandrosterone) positive blood test would be suggestive of an adrenal tumour as the underlying cause. Congenital adrenal hyperplasia (CAH) is a cause of this, see pg 116.
- Testicular feminization syndrome results when an XY individual develops a phenotypically female appearance as a result of the absence of testosterone receptors on end-organs. Serum testosterone levels are very high. A lack of testosterone receptors on the pituitary means that there can be no negative feedback leading to uninhibited release of gonadotrophin, leading to high LH and FSH levels.

Congenital adrenal hyperplasia
CAH
Cortisol low
Androgen high
Hairy

Topic facts

Congenital adrenal hyperplasia (CAH) is an autosomal recessive condition caused by enzyme defects in the steroid production pathway in the adrenals. The biochemical and physical findings are summarized in the memory aid.

- Most cases of CAH are caused by abnormalities of enzymes 11- and 21-hydroxylase.
- 21-Hydroxylase accounts for about 90 per cent of cases.
- Summary of steroid pathway:
  - steroid production starts with cholesterol
  - cholesterol is converted to form progesterone, testosterone, cortisol and aldosterone
  - enzyme abnormalities in CAH prevent production of cortisol and aldosterone, leading to a build-up of the precursors (progesterone and testosterone)
  - low levels of cortisol stimulate adrenocorticotrophic hormone (ACTH) release (through negative feedback), which compounds the problem, leading to production of more precursors that cannot be processed into cortisol or aldosterone.
- High levels of testosterone lead to precocious (early) puberty in men and ambiguous genitalia in women, as well as primary amenorrhoea, hirsuitism and virilism.
- Tests show a high ACTH, presence of urinary pregnanetriol and high level of 17-hydroxyprogesterone.
- Treatment is with cortisol replacement.

DiGeorge syndrome

Poor	little	George
Parathyroid	kids	Di**G**eorge syndrome

Topic facts

DiGeorge syndrome is a rare developmental defect of the pharyngeal pouches. There may be structural abnormalities of the parathyroid gland, thymus gland, aortic arch and face. The pathology and prognosis are summarized.

- DiGeorge syndrome is associated with a chromosome 22 abnormality.
- Newborn babies with parathyroid absence present with tetany (which can be fatal).
- Parathyroid hormone (PTH) maintains the level of Ca^{2+} in the blood. Lack of PTH leads to low levels of Ca^{2+} and consequently tetany occurs.
- Recall of the presenting features of DiGeorge syndrome aids understanding of parathyroid gland function and the role of Ca^{2+} in the blood.
- Muscle spasm occurs during hyperventilation. This results from low levels of ionized calcium caused by a disturbance in the balance of ionized calcium.
- Functional hypoparathyroidism is related to prolonged hypomagnesaemia. This is because magnesium is an important cofactor required for the release of PTH.
- Thymus gland involvement results in immune deficiency (typically T cell – risk of infection from encapsulated bacteria, viruses and fungi).

Diabetes insipidus
Head/Kidneys

Head (cranial)
- Trauma (injury/surgery – sphenoidal)
- Hypothalamic (pituitary tumour)
- Granulomas (sarcoidosis, histiocytosis)
- Infections (meningitis, encephalitis)
- Vascular (haemorrhage, thrombosis)
- Familial
- Idiopathic

Kidneys (nephrogenic)
- Drugs (lithium, glibenclamide)
- Metabolic (hyperkalaemia, hypercalcaemia, prolonged polyuria of any cause)
- Familial
- Renal tubular acidosis

Topic facts
Diabetes insipidus is a disorder of antidiuretic hormone (ADH) production/response, causes of which are given above.
- To differentiate between nephrogenic and cranial diabetes insipidus investigate with a fluid deprivation and desmopressin test.
- Cranial diabetes insipidus (CDI) will have a dilute urine sample (<300 mmol/kg), which will become concentrated (>800 mmol/kg) on administering desmopressin (a synthetic form of ADH).
- There will be no change in the urine concentration of nephrogenic diabetes insipidus (NDI) because the problem lies in the kidney, and blood levels of ADH are already high. Those with primary polydipsia will have a concentrated urine after fluid deprivation.

Diabetes-related skin disease

Get **A** **N**ew **L**eg

Granuloma **A**nnulare

Necrobiosis **L**ipoidica

Topic facts

The skin conditions commonly associated with diabetes mellitus are given above.

- Both can occur independently or present before the onset of diabetes.
- Both conditions have similar histological findings with necrosis of collagen.
- Both may regress spontaneously over a period of years.
- Necrobiosis lipoidica may be extensive and leave scarring.
- Whether good diabetic control improves healing remains controversial.
- No effective treatment has been found.
- The other important skin condition related to diabetes and insulin resistance is acanthosis nigricans (velvety-brown hyperpigmentation of the axilla and groin). This is also more common in overweight individuals.
- People with diabetes are also prone to skin infections when undiagnosed or if poorly controlled. The high sugar content allows bacteria to flourish. Patients may present with boils, furuncles or cellulitis.
- If there is vascular involvement, skin changes may be present in the lower limbs. Gangrene or arterial ulcers occur in severe cases.
- Arterial involvement is suggested by the presence of shiny, hairless, cool limbs with absence of peripheral pulses.

Hyperaldosteronism
Organ failure + **Conn's** syndrome and **Cushing's** syndrome

Organ failure
- Liver failure
- Heart failure
- Renal (nephrotic syndrome)

Conn's syndrome

Cushing's syndrome

Topic facts
Causes of hyperaldosteronism are categorized above.
- The renin–angiotensin–aldosterone system is central to the control of body Na^+ levels.
- Hyperaldosteronism leads to a salt-retaining state in which fluid overload subsequently occurs.
- The biochemical findings are of high Na^+, low K^+ (loss of Mg^{2+} and high serum bicarbonate may also result).
- Water follows salt distribution and thus salt excess leads to volume overload. This may, in turn, lead to hyponatraemia, as a result of excessive fluid retention causing haemodilution.
- An important principle when treating patients with hyperaldosteronism is to avoid intake of salt and fluids containing sodium, i.e. physiological or 0.9 per cent saline or dextrose saline. The body is unable to clear the salt because of its salt-retaining state, and this exacerbates fluid retention and may lead to cardiac failure.
- Cushing's syndrome can cause hyperaldosteronism as the excess corticosteroids have a weak mineralocorticoid effect.
- Hyperaldosteronism is a secondary cause of systemic hypertension (see page 33).
- Primary hyperaldosteronism may present with hyperglycaemia (low K^+ causes insulin suppression).

Hyperthyroidism

Got **T**oo **M**uch **T**hyroxine
Graves' disease
Toxic **M**ultinodular goitre
Toxic adenoma

Topic facts

The common causes of hyperthyroidism are given above.

- These three disorders account for most causes of hyperthyroidism.
- Clinical features of thyroid disease can be categorized into markers that indicate thyroid status (hyper-, hypo- or euthyroidism) and markers of thyroid disease.
- The indicators of thyroid status that should be assessed are pulse rate, rhythm (± atrial fibrillation), sweaty palms, fine tremor, restlessness, lid lag and thyroid bruits. Reflexes and voice (slow relaxing reflexes and a hoarse voice) indicate hypothyroidism. Most patients will be euthyroid. The most discriminating factor is pulse rate.
- Clinical markers of thyroid disease in hyperthyroidism include:
  - weight loss
  - gynaecomastia
  - amenorrhoea
  - diarrhoea
  - hair thinning
  - proximal myopathy
  - atrial fibrillation
  - osteoporosis
  - hypercalcaemia
  - eye signs in those with hyperthyroid Graves' disease.
- Exopthalmus occurs **o**nly in GRAVES' disease. Thyroid eye disease and the soft tissue signs (pretibial myxoedema and thyroid acropachy) are specific to Graves' disease.

Endocrinology

Hypogonadism
Acquired/Systemic/Primary

Acquired
- Pituitary disease:
  - Hypopituitarism
  - Haemochromatosis
  - Hyperprolactinaemia
- Oestrogen excess
- Drugs (anti-androgens, spironolactone)
- Orchitis

Systemic
- Malignancy
- Renal failure
- Liver failure
- Sickle cell

Primary
- Klinefelter syndrome (XXY)
- Myotonic dystrophy
- Testis (vanishing syndrome)
- Noonan's syndrome

Topic facts
The manifold causes of hypogonadism have been simplified and categorized with the more common ones listed here.
- Hypogonadism is the result of impairment of androgen levels.
- Phenotypic features of hypogonadism include loss of male distribution of body hair, feminine body fat distribution and gynaecomastia.
- Primary causes include Klinefelter syndrome in which the patient has an extra X chromosome. Klinefelter syndrome patients are typically tall with small testes and the phenotypic features listed above.
- Klinefelter syndrome patients may be XXYY.

McCune–Albright syndrome

PFG

Precocious puberty/**P**igmented lesions

Fibrous dysplasia

G protein abnormality

Topic facts

McCune–Albright syndrome is an activating G-protein disorder. The presentation and pathology are summarized above.

- G proteins are cell surface messengers that use cyclic adenosine monophosphate (cAMP) as an intracellular messenger.
- The result is hyperfunction of the endocrine glands during early development.
- The key clinical features are of precocious puberty (early onset puberty), pigmented lesions (café-au-lait spots) and fibrous dysplasia of the bone.
- Fibrous dysplasia most commonly affects the long bones, ribs and skull.
- Bone scanning can identify areas of fibrous dysplasia.

  Gland hyperfunction and clinical findings:
  - gonads: precocious puberty
  - growth hormone: acromegaly
  - adrenal gland: Cushing's disease
  - thyroid: hyperthyroidism
  - parathyroid: hyperparathyroidism.

- Investigations are primarily of endocrine function.
- As the gland hyperfunction is independent of central control, pituitary hormones are suppressed, i.e. precocious puberty is associated with raised FSH and LH levels and suppressed gonadotrophins.
- Hypertension may result from elevation of growth hormone levels.

Endocrinology

Organ-specific autoimmune disease
ROAST LP

Renal (renal tubular acidosis)
Ovarian (premature ovarian failure)
Adrenal (Addison's disease)
Stomach (pernicious anaemia, atrophic gastritis)
Thyroid (Graves' disease, myxoedema, Hashimoto's thyroiditis)
Liver (primary biliary cirrhosis)
Pancreas (diabetes mellitus)

Topic facts

The organ-specific autoimmune diseases are summarized in this topic.

- The organ-specific autoimmune diseases are a spectrum of autoimmune disease. Patients suffering from one type of organ-specific disease are at an increased risk of acquiring another.
- Other organ-specific autoimmune diseases not listed in the mnemonic are fibrosing alveolitis, chronic active hepatitis and idiopathic hypoparathyroidism.
- Vitiligo is a cutaneous marker of organ-specific autoimmune diseases (but also occurs independently).
- Schmidt's syndrome is one of the polyglandular autoimmune syndromes and is discussed on page 129.

Osteomalacia
Osteoma↓acia
> ↓ **Low vitamin D**
> ↓ **Low calcium**
> ↓ **Low phosphate**

Topic facts
This topic aids recall of the biochemical changes found in osteomalacia.

- Osteomalacia is commonly caused by vitamin D deficiency (but may also be the result of metabolic disorders). It is the adult version of rickets.
- The biochemical findings are, therefore, low vitamin D, low calcium and low phosphate. To remember this every time I write osteomalacia, I draw a downward arrow instead of an L.
- Alkaline phosphatase levels are raised as a result of calcium reabsorption from bones.
- The parathyroid hormone level is raised. This is the most sensitive marker of vitamin D deficiency.
- The underlying cause of the vitamin D deficiency may be the result of one of the following.

Malabsorption
- Small bowel disease, i.e. Crohn's disease
- Pancreatitis
- Gastrectomy

Inactive vitamin D
- Liver disease
- Phenytoin
- Chronic renal failure

Renal problems
- Nephrotic syndrome (loss of vitamin D-binding protein)
- Fanconi's syndrome

Endocrinology

Endocrinology

Phaeochromocytoma
The rule of 10 per cent
   10 per cent are bilateral
   10 per cent are malignant
   10 per cent are extra-adrenal
   10 per cent are familial

Topic facts
The rule of 10 per cent is a well-known rule of thumb relating to the presentation and pathology of phaeochromocytoma.
- The adrenal medulla is the only place in which the enzyme that converts norepinephrine (noradrenaline) to epinephrine (adrenaline) is found. Thus, phaeochromocytomas arising outside the adrenal medulla can release norepinephrine but not epinephrine.
- Familial phaeochromocytomas virtually all arise from the adrenal medulla.

Nobody **L**ikes **M**alignant **H**ypertension
   Neurofibromatosis
   Leiomyosarcoma (gastric)
   Multiple endocrine neoplasia
   von **H**ippel–Lindau syndrome

Topic facts
The diseases associated with phaeochromocytoma are given in this mnemonic.
- Phaeochromocytoma is found in multiple endocrine neoplasia (MEN) types 2a and 2b.
- Phaeochromocytoma is associated with neurofibromatosis type 1 (von Recklinghausen's disease).
- Phaeochromocytoma is a cause of malignant hypertension.

Polydipsia

Patients **K**eep **N**eeding **D**rink **C**onstantly

  Primary polydipsia
  Kidney failure
  Nephrogenic diabetes insipidus
  Dehydration/**D**rugs (lithium)/Diabetes mellitus
  Cranial diabetes insipidus/Calcium (raised)

Topic facts

Polydipsia is the high oral intake of fluid; the common causes are covered in this topic.

- Primary polydipsia is a psychiatric disorder in which the excessive intake of water leads to polyuria.
- Polyuria often accompanies polydipsia and is defined as the production of more than 3 L of dilute urine in 24 h.
- The polyuric phase of chronic renal failure can lead to polydipsia in an attempt to compensate for water loss.
- Dehydration may result from excessive fluid losses through the skin or loss through the kidneys. Kidney losses may be caused by diabetes insipidus, drug-induced polyuria (diuretics, lithium), hypercalcaemia or osmotic diuresis through hyperglycaemia in diabetes mellitus.
- Nephrogenic diabetes insipidus occurs as a result of resistance to the action of vasopressin on the kidneys.
- Drugs, particularly lithium, can induce a nephrogenic diabetes insipidus state.
- Cranial diabetes insipidus results from impaired ADH (vasopressin) secretion. Diabetes insipidus is discussed on page 118.
- Investigation is with urine volume, plasma biochemistry (in particular electrolytes) and osmolality in the serum and urine.
- Patients with normal blood tests go on to have a water deprivation test.
- Diabetes mellitus causes an osmotic diuresis and subsequent dehydration, hence thirst and polydipsia.

Endocrinology

Prolactin elevation

6 Ps

Pregnancy
Pill (oral contraceptive)
Polycystic ovary syndrome
Prolactinoma
Psychiatric drugs
Primary hypothyroidism

Endocrinology

Topic facts

This mnemonic lists the more common causes of hyperprolactinaemia.

- Prolactinoma is the most common hormone-secreting pituitary tumour.
- Large prolactinomas can lead to compression of the pituitary and secondary hypopituitarism.
- Coexistent bitemporal hemianopia indicates compression of the optic chiasm by the enlarged pituitary.
- Clinical features of hyperprolactinaemia are dependent on sex and age.
- Women of menstruating age present with amenorrhoea/oligomenorrhoea and galactorrhoea.
- Men complain of reduced libido, infertility and impotence.
- Dopamine agonists (bromocriptine) are used in the medical treatment of prolactinoma because they inhibit prolactin release.
- Primary hypothyroidism can cause hyperprolactinaemia as high levels of thyroid hormone-releasing hormone (TRH) stimulate prolactin production.
- Many of the psychiatric drugs are anti-dopaminergic and can result in hyperprolactinaemia. Examples include the phenothiazines, risperidone, olanzapine, amisulpiride and zotepine.

Schmidt's syndrome
TAD
Thyroid (Hashimoto's Thyroiditis)
Adrenal (Addison's disease)
Diabetes mellitus

Topic facts
Schmidt's syndrome is a polyglandular autoimmune disease. The autoimmune diseases that make up Schmidt's syndrome are given here.

- The polyglandular autoimmune diseases (PGADs) are groups of organ-specific autoimmune disease that typically present together.
- There are three types of PGAD, termed type 1, type 2 (Schmidt's syndrome) and type 3.
- Type 2 is the most common and is the combination of autoimmune disease affecting the thyroid, adrenals and pancreas.
- The adrenals are often the first organ affected in type 2 PGAD.
- Type 1 is rare, and mainly affects children with involvement of the adrenals and parathyroids.
- Type 3 involves the thyroid and other autoimmune diseases without involvement of the adrenals.
- Candidates should be aware of the triad that makes up Schmidt's syndrome but are unlikely to be asked questions involving the other types.

Endocrinology

Stress hormones
GET C
Glucagon/**G**rowth hormone
Epinephrine (adrenaline)
Thyroxine
Cortisol

Topic facts
The hormones that make up the stress response are given in this topic.
- The hormones released by the body when under stress all have an anti-insulin-like action.
- Think of insulin as a 'relaxed' hormone: levels rise as we sit back and digest our food after a meal.
- It is helpful to remember this when performing hormone suppression tests.
- Examples are given below:
  - a good example is the investigation of acromegaly with the oral glucose tolerance test. A glucose load will lead to a rise in insulin levels and a suppression of the stress hormones. A normal individual will suppress his or her growth hormone level to <1–2 mIU/L. People with acromegaly fail to suppress growth hormone and may have a paradoxical rise in growth hormone levels.
  - another example is the use of the insulin tolerance test for growth hormone reserve. Insulin is administered after an overnight fast. Hypoglycaemia is induced and the stress hormones respond, including growth hormone. Levels are expected to exceed 20 mIU/L. Cortisol levels should rise by at least 180 from basal levels.

Thyroid cancer
PFAM

Papillary
Follicular
Anaplastic
Medullary

Topic facts
The causes of thyroid cancer in order of most common occurrence are summarized above.

- Papillary carcinoma:
  - the most common form of thyroid cancer; it is more common in women and it presents between the ages of 20 and 50 years
  - most patients present with a non-tender palpable nodule
  - investigation is with fine-needle aspiration and ultrasonography of the thyroid
  - prognosis is good.
- Follicular carcinoma:
  - the second most common type
  - the peak age of presentation is around 50 years (but can present earlier) and is more common in women
  - prognosis is less good than papillary carcinoma but still favourable.
- Anaplastic thyroid cancer:
  - a disease of elderly people – typically women aged over 60 years
  - patients present with a rapidly enlarging mass in the neck; survival after diagnosis for most is several months as the disease spreads rapidly.
- Medullary carcinoma:
  - found in MEN types 2a and 2b.

Renal

- Lipoatrophy
- Nephritic syndrome
- Nephrotoxic drugs
- Renally excreted drugs
- Renal failure (acute)
- Renal failure (chronic)
- Renal failure and large kidneys
- Rhabdomyolysis

Lipoatrophy
Protruding **M**uscles
   Protease inhibitors
   Mesangiocapillary glomerulonephritis (MACGN)

Topic facts
Lipoatrophy is the loss of normal fat deposition. The two common causes are protease inhibitors and MACGN.

- Lipoatrophy exposes the underlying facial musculature, which results in an angular, masculine-looking facial appearance.
- HIV patients on protease inhibitors may demonstrate this change as a side effect of their treatment.
- Look specifically for lipoatrophy in renal failure patients because this will give you the underlying diagnosis and impress your examiners.
- Clues to patients with renal failure:
  - scars from old fistulas
  - active fistulas with a venous hum
  - gum hypertrophy and hairiness resulting from use of ciclosporin immunosuppressant
  - J-shaped abdominal scars and masses in the iliac fossa from renal transplantations.
- Clues to the underlying cause of renal failure:
  - lipoatrophy and MACGN
  - blood glucose monitoring charts, blood glucose needle marks on the fingers, insulin pens, granuloma annulare, necrobiosis lipoidica – diabetes mellitus
  - blood pressure charts or antihypertensive medication in the hypertensive patient.
- Side-effects of immunosuppressants are a common question in Part 2 and PACES. Be aware of the commonly used drugs – azathioprine, ciclosporin and tacrolimus – and their side-effects.

Renal

Nephritic syndrome
High **P**rotein **O**utput
   Haematuria/**H**ypertension
   Proteinuria (<2 g/day)
   Oedema/**O**liguria

Topic facts
The clinical findings that present in nephritic syndrome are given in this memory aid.

- Nephritic syndrome is most commonly secondary to a streptococcal infection that the patient may have had 1–3 weeks before presentation.
- It is also associated with systemic lupus erythematosus (SLE).
- SLE nephritis has a so-called 'full house' immunostaining picture. On staining, IgG, IgM, IgA and complement are all present – a full house of the immune system.
- Investigations:
  - baseline renal function
  - creatinine clearance, 24-hour protein excretion or albumin:creatinine ratio.
- Diagnostically useful tests:
  - urine microscopy for red cell casts (indicative of glomerulonephritis)
  - throat and skin cultures and serum antistreptolysin O titre (ASOT) – helpful in diagnosing recent streptococcal infection
  - ANAs (anti-nuclear antibodies) and anti-DNA anti bodies are useful in the diagnosis of SLE
  - C3 nephritic factor helps diagnose mesangiocapillary glomerulonephritis
  - ANCA (anti-neutrophil cytoplasmic antibody) for Wegener's granulomatosis – suspect this if there is a history of respiratory problems or chest radiograph showing cavities.

Nephrotoxic drugs

Nephrotoxic **D**rugs **A**re **C**ommonly **G**iven

NSAIDs
Diuretics (bendrofluazide)
Aminoglycosides
Ciclosporin
Gold

Topic facts

Commonly used nephrotoxic drugs are shown above.

- Many of the commonly used drugs are nephrotoxic. It is important to be aware of the more common ones in order to avoid, or dose adjust, in renal impairment.
- The cause of renal damage differs but can be broadly divided into three categories: drugs that cause direct toxicity to the renal tubules, drugs that cause ischaemia through impairment of renal perfusion and drugs that cause glomerulonephritis.
- Aminoglycosides cause direct toxicity and are one of the most commonly used drugs in this category. Dosage should be adjusted on the basis of serum drug levels. They should be used in caution in patients with renal impairment.
- NSAIDs impair renal perfusion through afferent vasoconstriction. Angiotensin-converting enzyme (ACE) inhibitors cause efferent arteriolar dilation. The two effects combine to reverse the natural bottle-neck required to provide the filtration pressure necessary to maintain an adequate glomerular filtration rate. Ischaemia followed by acute tubular necrosis develops.
- Ciclosporin, an immunosuppressant, also causes vasoconstriction, which can lead to acute renal failure. (Ciclosporin induces chronic renal failure through degenerative changes.)
- Gold is a cause of glomerulonephritis.

Renal

Renally excreted drugs
DAMP
Digoxin/**D**iuretics
Aspirin/**A**minoglycosides
Metformin/**M**ethotrexate
Penicillin/**P**robenecid

Topic facts
Common renally excreted drugs are given here.
- Failure to excrete drugs can lead to complications as a result of:
  - raised serum levels resulting in toxic effects
  - toxic metabolites of the drug
  - impaired drug efficacy in those with renal impairment.
- Dose adjustment advice is given in Appendix 3 – renal impairment – of the *British National Formulary* (or online at www.bnf.org). A basic summary is included below.
- Total dose can be adjusted by reducing either dose quantity or dose frequency.
- A loading dose is often required if the maintenance dose is reduced (because, in renal impairment, the half-life of renally excreted drugs is prolonged, and this delays the time that it takes for a drug to reach the therapeutic steady-state plasma concentration. The loading dose is typically the same as the normal first dose for patients without renal impairment).
- Water-soluble drugs are cleared through glomerular filtration. Other drugs are cleared through active tubular secretion; examples include loop diuretics, NSAIDs and metformin.
- Metformin should be avoided in type 2 diabetics with renal impairment, because of the risk of lactic acidosis.

Renal failure (acute)
Prerenal/Intrinsic/Postrenal

Prerenal (hypovolaemia)
- Bleeding, burns, diarrhoea, pancreatitis, diuretics, sepsis
- Poor cardiac output (myocardial infarct, heart failure, massive pulmonary embolus)
- Clots (renal artery/vein thrombosis)

Intrinsic (Is Always Vasculitis)
- **I**nterstitial nephritis (allergy, infection)
- **A**cute tubular necrosis (ATN) (ischaemia, toxins)
- **V**asculitis and glomerulonephritis (Wegener's granulomatosis, Goodpasture's syndrome)

Postrenal (obstruction)
- Urinary tract obstruction

Topic facts
The common causes of acute renal failure are summarized here.
- There are many causes of acute renal failure. Prerenal causes are by far the most common.
- Prerenal renal failure results from inadequate perfusion of the kidneys.
- Intrinsic renal failure results from damage to the kidneys directly.
- Hypovolaemia and ATN represent a continuum, i.e. patients with severe hypovolaemia, if left long enough, develop ATN secondary to ischaemia.
- ATN can also be caused by toxins (bacterial toxins, Bence Jones protein, gentamicin).
- Vasculitis and glomerulonephritis are the second most common cause of acute renal failure.

Renal

Renal failure (chronic)
He **G**ets **V**ery **T**ired

Hereditary
- Polycystic kidney disease

Glomerular disease
- Primary
- Secondary (diabetes mellitus, SLE, amyloid)

Vascular disease
- Hypertension
- Atheroma
- Vasculitis

Tubulointerstitial disease
- Reflux/pyelonephritis
- Nephrocalcinosis
- Interstitial nephritis
- Obstruction

Topic facts
Lethargy is a common presenting symptom in patients with chronic renal failure, causes of which are summarized above.

- Diabetes, chronic glomerulonephritis and hypertension are the most common causes of chronic renal failure in the UK.
- Findings in favour of chronic renal failure include small kidneys, normocytic anaemia and uraemia, which is well tolerated.
- Patients present complaining of lethargy, pruritis, fluid retention and shortness of breath.
- Adult polycystic kidney disease (APCKD) is discussed on pages 88 and 139.

Renal failure and large kidneys

Huge **C**(k)idneys **A**re **D**amaged

    Hydronephrosis/**H**ypertrophy

    Clots

    Amyloidosis/**A**cromegaly/**A**PCKD

    Diabetic nephropathy (early)

Topic facts

This mnemonic lists the causes of renal impairment and large kidneys.

- Hydronephrosis is the most common cause of renal impairment and renal enlargement.
- Hypertrophy of a single functioning kidney may lead to a unilateral palpable renal mass.
- 'Clots' refers to acute renal vein thrombosis. This results in a tense, enlarged kidney. Patients present with flank pain, nausea, vomiting and haematuria.
- Amyloid deposits in the kidneys and liver lead to enlargement of these organs. Amyloid is identified histologically with the use of Congo red to which amyloid stains apple-green.
- Acromegaly causes soft tissue hypertrophy and thus renal enlargement.
- APCKD is an autosomal dominant condition in which cysts form in the kidneys and other organs. It is associated with renal failure and uni- or bilateral renal enlargement.
- In the early stages of diabetic nephropathy there is renal enlargement.

Renal

Rhabdomyolysis

Electrocution **S**everely **N**ecroses **M**uscles

Electrocution

Statins/**S**epsis/**S**eizure/**S**tasis

Neuroleptic malignant syndrome

Marathon runners

Topic facts

Rhabdomyolysis is the breakdown of skeletal muscle with the release of myoglobin into the blood.

- Myoglobin is extremely nephrotoxic and can lead to acute renal failure.
- Damaged cells leak potassium, phosphate and creatinine kinase. High levels of these are seen on blood tests.
- A positive urine dipstick test for blood in the absence of red blood cells on urine microscopy is a useful test for myoglobinuria (urine dipsticks cannot differentiate between haemoglobin and myoglobin).
- The mainstay of treatment is hydration and management of hyperkalaemia.
- Those with very high creatinine kinase levels may benefit from alkalinization of the urine, to help increase solubility of the myoglobin.
- Diuretics may be used in patients with poor urine output despite adequate rehydration to promote diuresis.
- Stasis refers to patients who fall and lie undetected for an extended period of time. The elderly are at greatest risk of this cause.

Respiratory

- Bilateral hilar lymphadenopathy
- Bronchial carcinoma
- Bronchiectasis
- Collapsed lung
- Consolidation
- Cor Pulmonale
- Cyanosis
- Empyema
- Haemoptysis
- Obstructive airways disease
- Pleural effusion
- Pneumothorax
- Pulmonary fibrosis
- Pulmonary hypertension
- Respiratory failure
- Yellow-nail syndrome

Bilateral hilar lymphadenopathy

Mediastinal **L**ymphadenopathy **T**ypically **S**arcoid
> **M**alignancy
> **L**ymphoma
> **T**uberculosis (TB)
> **S**arcoid

Topic facts

This mnemonic summarizes common causes of bilateral hilar lymphadenopathy (BHL).

- Sarcoidosis and lymphoma are the most common causes of BHL.
- Bronchial (or other) neoplasm with metastasis to the mediastinal lymph nodes can lead to bilateral hilar enlargement. Look for evidence of a primary source (history of weight loss, prior cancer).
- Lymphoma patients may have evidence of lymphadenopathy elsewhere (± hepatospienomegaly).
- TB is suggested by a history of exposure to risk factors, e.g. contact with infected individuals, those living in institutions (prisons), foreign travel.
- Sarcoidosis is a multisystem granulomatous disorder. The lung is most commonly affected but other organs are often involved.
  - patients may present with Löfgren's syndrome:
    - erythema nodosum
    - BHL
    - arthralgia
    - anterior uveitis.
  - hypercalcaemia may be present. The granulomas lead to the production of activated vitamin D.
  - disease course may be monitored using serum ACE levels (these are not diagnostic because they can be elevated in a number of conditions).
  - sarcoid is more common in females and those of African–Caribbean origin.

Bronchial carcinoma

Types
SOLA
- **S**quamous
- **O**at cell
- **L**arge cell
- **A**denocarcinoma

Complications
High **DOMES**
- **H**orner's syndrome (sympathetic nerve compression)
- **H**oarse voice (recurrent laryngeal nerve compression)
- **H**igh diaphragm (phrenic nerve compression)

- **D**irect spread (Pancoast's tumour)
- **O**bstruction of bronchus
- **M**alignant pleural effusion
- **E**rosion of large vessel
- **S**VC (superior vena cava) obstruction

Topic facts
The first mnemonic is well known and lists the types of lung cancer in order of most common occurrence. The second lists the complications associated with bronchial neoplasm (high domes refers to diaphragmatic elevation caused by phrenic nerve involvement).

- Lung cancer is the second most common cancer in the UK (after breast) and prognosis is poor.
- Important predisposing factors include smoking, asbestos exposure and atmospheric pollution.

Respiratory

Bronchiectasis

He **K**eeps **O**n **C**oughing **I**nfected **C**rap

Hypogammaglobulinaemia
Kartagener's syndrome
Obstruction: foreign body
Cystic fibrosis
Infection: measles, pertussis in children, bronchiolitis of infancy
Cancer: lymphadenopathy

Topic facts

Bronchiectasis is the chronic dilatation of the bronchial tree complicated by impaired clearance of bronchial secretions and infection. Causes are given in the mnemonic above.

- Infectious causes of bronchiectasis are commonly caused by *Haemophilus influenzae*.
- Consider bronchiectasis in a patient with clubbing and coarse crackles (the differential of clubbing and crackles is bronchiectasis, bronchial neoplasm and fibrosing alveolitis).
- Identifying cystic fibrotic patients:
  - bedside clues such as a sputum pot or creon tablets
  - inspection:
    - cystic fibrotic patients may be short and underweight as a result of malabsorption
    - tunnelled lines with ports palpable under the skin, for injection of antibiotics, in patients with recurrent infection.
- Kartagener's syndrome is the result of cilial dysmotility and is associated with dextrocardia and infertility.

Respiratory

Collapsed lung

Often **P**neumothorax

Obstruction:
- Foreign body
- Cancer
- Clot
- Mucus
- Lymphadenopathy

Pneumothorax/**P**leural effusion

Topic facts

This topic lists the causes of a collapsed lung.
- There are three main causes of lung collapse: pneumothorax, pleural effusion and obstruction.
- Pneumothorax (not tension) and obstruction both lead to loss of volume on the affected side. Identify:
  - reduced expansion on inspection
  - reduced expansion on palpation (the upper lobes are assessed primarily at the front of the chest and expand mainly anteroposteriorly; compare the degree of lift between both hands; the lower lobes are best assessed from the back and expand laterally; compare the degree of separation of the hands)
  - hyperresonant to percussion
  - tracheal deviation towards the affected side
  - tracheal and apex beat deviation away from the affected side may occur in large pneumothorax
  - reduced breath may sounds on affected side
- Very large pleural effusions push the trachea away from the affected side and are stony dull (see page 152).
- Look for associated signs, e.g. clubbing, lymphadenopathy, marfanoid features.

Respiratory

Consolidation
PIC
Pulmonary infarction
Infection
Carcinoma

Topic facts
The causes of consolidation are summarized above.
- Consolidation is most commonly due to an infective process.
- The key clinical features of consolidation are:
  - dullness to percussion
  - crackles
  - increased vocal resonance and tactile vocal fremitus
  - bronchial breath sounds.
- Common community-acquired organisms of infection in order of most common presentation are:
  - *Streptococcus pneumoniae*
  - *Mycoplasma pneumoniae*
  - *Haemophilus influenzae*
  - *Legionella* sp.
  - *Chlamydia* sp.
  - *Staphylococcus aureus*
  - *Klebsiella* sp.
  - mycobacteria (TB).
- Lung cancer can present as consolidation with infective consolidation distal to where the tumour lies within the bronchial tree causing a partial obstruction. There may be an associated wheeze, which is characteristically monophonic.
- Pulmonary infarction may be associated with a pleural rub. Clinical features suggestive of this include haemoptysis, pleuritic pain and the presence of a small pleural effusion.

Cor Pulmonale

Cor **P**ulmonale **F**requently **E**mphysema
   Chronic obstructive pulmonary disease (COPD)
   Primary pulmonary hypertension (PPH)
   Fibrosis
   Emboli

Topic facts

Cor pulmonale is defined as right-sided heart failure secondary to pulmonary pathology. Common causes are given here.

- The mechanism of right heart failure in cor pulmonale is increased pulmonary vascular resistance.
- COPD is the most common cause of cor pulmonale.
- In the case of chronic pulmonary disease, inadequate ventilation in the affected area results in hypoxia, induced vasoconstriction and subsequent pulmonary hypertension.
- Multiple pulmonary emboli increase pulmonary vascular resistance as a result of vessel obstruction by the emboli.
- Examination of a patient with right heart failure should include a respiratory examination to assess for cor pulmonale.
- PPH is uncommon and secondary causes of pulmonary hypertension should be excluded.
- PPH is more common in young women and is associated with the connective tissue diseases.
- Shortness of breath is the most common presenting symptom of PPH.
- Investigation for PPH should include autoantibodies, chest radiograph and echocardiogram.
- PPH treatment includes anticoagulation and the use of vasodilators and prostaglandins.

Cyanosis

Very **C**onstricted **A**rteries
Significantly **A**lter **H**and **C**olour

Peripheral

Vasoconstriction (Raynaud's phenomenon)
Cardiac output low (heart failure, aortic stenosis)
Arterial occlusion (atheroma)

Central

Shunt (right-to-left cardiac shunt)
Altitude (low Po_2 of air at high altitude)
Hypoventilation
Cor pulmonale

Topic facts

This topic identifies the causes of cyanosis, categorized by location.

- A minimum of 5 g deoxygenated haemoglobin is required to identify cyanosis clinically. An approximate haemoglobin level of 8 g/dL is required to achieve an arterial blood gas (ABG) oxygen level of 8. This means that, unless the patient is polycythaemic, he or she will be in, or close to, type 1 respiratory failure.
  - for example, a patient with a haemoglobin of 13 g/dL is cyanosed. This means at least 5 g of the haemoglobin is deoxygenated: $13 - 5 = 8$. This leaves 8 g oxygenated haemoglobin. The patient will therefore be in borderline type 1 respiratory failure.
- Beware of the blood gas that shows a normal Po_2 level in the patient gasping for breath. ABGs simply measure gas transfer from lungs into plasma. Patients may die of hypoxia with a 'normal ABG Po_2' if there is no Hb to bind the available O_2 as a result of anaemia.

Empyema

My **L**ung **S**ecretes **P**us
   Mediastinal sepsis
   Lung abscess
   Surgery/**S**ubphrenic abscess
   Pneumonia (TB)

Topic facts

Empyema is defined as pus inside the pleural cavity, the causes of which are summarized here.

- Empyema is most commonly secondary to bacterial infection. A pleural effusion forms and in some cases then progresses to form a loculated pus-filled cavity.
- Empyema is associated with high morbidity and mortality (up to 20 per cent in the most severe cases).
- The most common causative organisms are *Staphylococcus aureus* and anaerobes.
- Empyema development can be avoided by the recognition and treatment of bacterial pneumonia with antibiotics. Those with effusions are at most risk.
- Chest radiograph remains the first-line investigation to confirm the presence of pleural fluid.
- Ultrasonography of the chest is useful to identify smaller volumes of fluid, the presence of loculated effusions and the marking of sites for drainage.
- Computed tomography (CT) of the thorax is the most diagnostically useful imaging modality because it can best identify the presence of empyema and any coexistent infection.
- Prognosticators of a poor outcome:
  - pH of pleural fluid <7.2 (indicative of empyema)
  - large effusion
  - purulent pleural fluid
  - positive culture or Gram stain
  - presence of loculations.
- Patients with the above require chest drain ± fibrinolytic therapy. Severe cases require surgery.

Haemoptysis

Bloody **C**ough, **T**hink **PE M**aybe **L**VF

Bronchiectasis

Cancer (lung)

Tuberculosis (TB)

Pneumonia/**P**ulmonary embolism (PE)

Mitral stenosis

Left ventricular failure (LVF)

Topic facts

Haemoptysis is the production of blood-stained mucus; the common causes are given in the mnemonic above.

- Massive haemoptysis is more common in carcinoma but can also occur in bronchiectasis and pulmonary TB.
- Moderate haemoptysis occurs in pneumonia, mitral stenosis, PE and LVF.
- Rarer causes of haemoptysis to be considered include Goodpasture's syndrome, Wegener's granulomatosis and arteriovenous malformation.
- First-line investigation should include: chest radiograph for evidence of mass, or the presence of a wedge-shaped opacity in PE (rare). ECG to look for sinus tachycardia and right heart strain (suggestive of PE – the S1Q3T3 pattern is rare). D-dimer (if negative, probability of embolism is low). Erythrocyte sedimentation rate (ESR) – for evidence of vasculitis.
- If there is a high suspicion of a large PE, an urgent echocardiogram may show evidence of right heart strain as a result of sudden increase in pulmonary vascular resistance.
- Wegener's granulomatosis vasculitic findings – high ESR, rhinitis and renal involvement.
- Haemopytsis should be differentiated from swallowed epistaxis, haematemesis and blood from oral lesions.

Obstructive airway disease
ABCDE
  Asthma
  Bronchitis
  Chronic obstructive pulmonary disease
  Don't forget
  Emphysema

Topic facts
The causes of obstructive airway disease are summarized here.
- COPD encompasses both chronic bronchitis and emphysema.
- The most common cause of COPD is smoking-related disease.
- Acute asthma causes reversible airway obstruction.
- People with chronic asthma can develop a chronic obstructive picture as the disease progresses.
- Young patients and non-smokers with COPD should make the candidate suspicious of α_1-antitrypsin deficiency.
- COPD patients feature frequently in PACES because they are often in hospital, have clinical signs and are easy to get hold of. Most candidates will reach the diagnosis, and so to score highly one must examine slickly, demonstrating the clinical features and identifying the associated findings.
- Ensure you look for:
  - nicotine staining
  - clubbing
  - carbon dioxide retention flap
  - purpura from steroid usage
  - signs of neoplasm
  - cachexia
  - peripheral oedema and loud second heart sound in the patient with cor pulmonale.

Respiratory

Pleural effusion

Exudate
MRS SIP

    Malignant effusion
    Rheumatoid arthritis
    SLE
    Subphrenic abscess
    Infection (pneumonia, TB)
    Pulmonary embolism

Transudate
Cause **N**ot **L**ocal

    Cardiac failure
    Nephrotic syndrome
    Liver disease

Topic facts
Pleural effusion causes of are categorized here into exudate and transudate.
- A bloody tap is suggestive of malignancy but also occurs in large pulmonary emboli and TB infection.
- If mesothelioma is suspected, a pleural biopsy should be performed at the same time as a chest drain is inserted.
- A history of asbestos exposure and pleural calcification is consistent with mesothelioma.
- Pleural fluid should be sent for:
  - protein
  - glucose
  - pH
  - cytology
  - culture
  - Gram stain.

Pneumothorax
SIT
Spontaneous
- Chronic lung disease (COPD, asthma, bullae, pneumoconiosis)

Iatrogenic
- Surgery
- Thoracocentesis
- Central line needlesticks

Traumatic
- Rib fracture
- Stabbing

Topic facts
Pneumothorax is the presence of air in the pleural cavity; the causes are given above.

- Spontaneous pneumothorax without underlying lung disease is most common in young adults.
- The most common symptoms are chest pain and shortness of breath.
- Patients who delay before presenting to hospital are at an increased risk of pulmonary oedema on re-expansion of the collapsed lung.
- Investigation of choice is chest radiograph.
- ABG should be performed if the oxygen saturation is <93 per cent or if there is evidence of respiratory distress.
- Management involves needle aspiration and repeat radiograph. If this fails at the first attempt it should be repeated. If this fails a second time a chest drain should be inserted
- There is a 10–15 per cent chance of recurrence within 1 year of diagnosis of spontaneous pneumothorax.

Respiratory

Pulmonary fibrosis
BREAST CRASH

Upper
Bronchopulmonary aspergillosis (allergic)
Radiation
Extrinsic allergic alveolitis
Ankylosing spondylitis
Sarcoid
Tuberculosis

Lower
Cryptogenic fibrosis
Rheumatoid lung disease
Asbestos-related fibrosis
Systemic sclerosis
High-dose radiation

Topic facts
The causes of pulmonary fibrosis are categorized here by the common site of involvement.
- By dividing the causes of lung fibrosis into those of the upper and lower zones you can rapidly halve your list of causes and suggest the most appropriate diagnosis, based on age, sex and any coexisting clinical clues, for example:
  - peripheral deforming arthropathy: rheumatoid lung (the presence of rheumatoid nodules confirms the diagnosis of rheumatoid changes; lung involvement occurs in 2 per cent of rheumatoid cases)
  - chest tattoo dot: radiation-induced fibrosis
  - poor chest expansion and question mark posture: ankylosing spondylitis
  - cachexia (? Asian), with apical fibrosis: TB.

Pulmonary hypertension

Pulmonary **H**ypertension **C**auses **R**evealed

    Primary pulmonary hypertension (PPH)

    Hypoventilation

    COPD

    Cardiac causes (mitral valve disease, atrial septal defect/ventricular septal defect)

    Recurrent pulmonary emboli

Topic facts

The causes of pulmonary hypertension are summarized in this topic.

- Pulmonary hypertension is classified into primary and secondary causes.
- Secondary pulmonary hypertension is by far the most common type.
- COPD accounts for most cases of secondary pulmonary hypertension.
- Other important causes include recurrent pulmonary emboli, cardiac causes and hypoventilation (resulting from obstructive sleep apnoea, myopathies and obesity – Pickwickian syndrome).
- PPH is much less common and associated with a poor prognosis.
  - patients are typically young women who present with progressive shortness of breath on exercise.
  - PPH may occur independently but is associated with connective tissue diseases, vasculitis and HIV infection.
  - shortness of breath is the most common presenting symptom.
  - the management of PPH is discussed on page 147.

Respiratory

Respiratory failure

Type 1
A Low P_{O_2}
  Asthma
  Left ventricular failure
  Pulmonary embolus

Type 2
Hypoventilation

- COPD
- Severe asthma (patient tiring).
- Muscle weakness, e.g. Guillain–Barré syndrome
- Respiratory centre depression, e.g. with sedatives
- Chest wall deformities

Topic facts

Causes of type 1 and type 2 respiratory failure are summarized here.

- Type 1 respiratory failure is defined as a $P_{O_2} < 8$ kPa.
- Type 2 failure is defined as a $P_{O_2} < 8$ kPa and $P_{CO_2} > 6$ kPa.
- Type 1 failure occurs as a result of either impairment of gas transfer in the alveoli (pneumonia, pulmonary oedema, pulmonary embolus, fibrosing alveolitis) or right-to-left cardiac shunt.
- The most common cause of type 1 failure is asthma.
- Type 2 failure occurs as a result of hypoventilation; patients are unable to 'blow off' their waste CO_2.
- The most common cause of type 2 failure is COPD.
- Note that asthma can also cause type 2 respiratory failure when the patient becomes tired and is unable to ventilate the lungs adequately.

Yellow-nail syndrome
Lung + Lymphatics

Lung disease
- Bronchiectasis
- Pleural effusions
- COPD
- Lung cancer

Lymphatic hypoplasia
- Lymphoedema

Topic facts
Yellow-nail syndrome is a disorder that is characterized by the presence of thick, longitudinally and laterally curved yellow nails, which are slow growing. The findings associated with yellow-nail syndrome are given here.
- The fingertips are often exposed as a result of the slow growth and all nails are affected.
- Presentation occurs in middle-age.
- The importance of yellow-nail syndrome is primarily its association with lung disease (bronchiectasis, pleural effusions, COPD and lung cancer) and lymphatic hypoplasia, which presents as lymphoedema.

Rheumatology

- Ankylosing spondylitis
- Chondrocalcinosis
- Collagen diseases
- Connective tissue diseases
- Monoarthritis
- Psoriatic arthritis
- Raynaud's phenomenon
- Reiter's syndrome
- Rheumatoid arthritis
- Seronegative arthritis
- Vasculitis

Ankylosing spondylitis
Commonly known as the **A** disease

Anterior uveitis

Atlantoaxial subluxation

Apical fibrosis

Aortic regurgitation

Aortitis

Atrioventricular block

Arthritis

Arachnoiditis (spinal)

Amyloidosis

Achilles' tendonitis

Topic facts
Ankylosing spondylitis is commonly known as the A disease because the complications associated with it all begin with the letter A, as shown here.

- Ankylosing spondylitis is one of the HLA-B27-linked diseases. The HLA-B27 conditions include psoriatic arthritis, enteropathic arthritis and Reiter's syndrome.
- Presentation occurs in young to middle-aged adults.
- Anterior uveitis is the most common associated finding.
- Aortitis presents in 4 per cent of cases with features of aortic regurgitation.
- Schoeber's test is a clinical examination technique required for the assessment of ankylosing spondylitis. Look for the sacral dimples and mark 10 cm above and 5 cm below. Ask the patient to lean forwards and touch the toes. Measure the increase in distance between the two marks. A value <5 cm is associated with ankylosing spondylitis.
- Other associated features include IgA nephropathy and plantar fasciitis.

Chondrocalcinosis
WHAT GP
Wilson's disease
Haemochromatosis
Acromegaly
Thyroid (hypo-)
Gout
Parathyroid (hyper-)/**P**hosphate (hypo-)

Topic facts
Chondrocalcinosis is the calcification of cartilage, causes of which are given above.

- Chondrocalcinosis is often asymptomatic and found incidentally on radiographs; however, it can mimic osteoarthritis.
- Chondrocalcinosis can present as an acute swollen joint and in this case should be investigated with needle aspiration using a polarizing microscope. The presence of crystals suggests either:
  - calcium pyrophosphate (pseudogout) – positively birefringent or
  - gout – negatively birefringent.
- Chondrocalcinosis typically affects the large joints and, in particular, the knee.
- In elderly people a form of chrondrocalcinosis occurs as a result of deposition of calcium pyrophosphate in the cartilage.
- In most cases no cause is found.
- Renal patients on dialysis are prone to chondrocalcinosis.
- Treatment of chrondrocalcinosis is symptomatic with use of analgesia and rest. Acute cases require joint aspiration and investigation as for an acute swollen joint.

Collagen diseases
POEM
Pseudoxanthoma elasticum
Osteogenesis imperfecta
Ehlers–Danlos syndrome
Marfan syndrome

Topic facts
The collagen diseases are summarized in this topic.
- The collagen diseases are associated with blue sclerae on examination. They are common MRCP cases in the clinical examination.
- This group of disorders is associated with gastrointestinal bleeding as a result of increased fragility of the blood vessels.
- Mitral valve prolapse is a complication common to the collagen diseases.
- Pseudoxanthoma elasticum is an inherited collagen disorder associated with a defect of elastin. Inheritance may be dominant or recessive depending on the genetic abnormality.
- Clinical findings are of:
  - angioid streaks on the retina – dark streaks that radiate outwards from the optic disc
  - plucked chicken-skin appearance – typically found on the neck
  - increased skin elasticity – test by pulling out folds at the neck and axilla.
- Pseudoxanthoma elasticum patients develop vascular disease (vaso-occlusive arteriopathy) and are at increased risk of both coronary artery and peripheral vascular disease.
- Osteogenesis imperfecta patients are short, with skeletal deformities resulting from multiple fractures.
- Patients with Ehlers–Danlos syndrome present with bruising, scars, hyperflexible joints and increased skin laxity. Aortic dissection is an important complication.
- Marfan syndrome is discussed on pages 36 and 38.

Connective tissue diseases
MRS PD
Mixed connective tissue disease
Rheumatoid arthritis
Scleroderma/**S**LE (systemic lupus erythematosus)/**S**jögren's syndrome
Polyarteritis nodosa (PAN)
Dermatomyositis

Topic facts
The group of diseases that make up connective tissue diseases are summarized here.

- The connective tissue diseases are a spectrum of disorders. Patients with one connective tissue disease are at increased risk of developing another, so when one of these diseases is present you should look for features of the associated disorders.
- Mixed connective tissue disease is rare; presentation occurs in late teens to early 20s and pulmonary hypertension is the most common cause of death.
- The most common findings are Raynaud's phenomenon and arthritis, followed by swallowing difficulties and pulmonary involvement. Approximately half will develop the typical heliotropic rash.
- Investigations for connective tissue diseases:
  - ANA (anti-nuclear antibody): found in SLE, scleroderma, Sjögren's syndrome, mixed connective tissue disease and polymyositis
  - anti-Ro and -La: Sjögren's syndrome
  - anti-smooth muscle: SLE (very specific)
  - anti-dsDNA: SLE (specific)
  - anti-Jo: polymyositis
  - anti-Scl: systemic sclerosis
  - anti-centromere: CREST (**c**alcinosis, **R**aynaud's phenomenon, o**e**sophagitis, **s**clerosis, **t**elangiectasia)
  - anti-RNP (antibody to ribonucleoprotein): mixed connective tissue disease, SLE.

Monoarthritis

Osteoarthritis **G**ives **S**evere **P**ain

    Osteoarthritis

    Gout

    Septic arthritis

    Pseudogout

Topic facts

Monoarthritis is the inflammation of a single joint; the common causes are covered here.

- Rarer causes of monoarthritis include:
  - rheumatoid arthritis
  - spondyloarthropathies
  - tuberculosis infection
  - haemarthrosis (haemophilia).
- Trauma should also be considered as a cause, although this is usually apparent in the history and clinical examination.
- Joint aspiration is the most diagnostically useful test in the acute swollen joint. It can help differentiate sepsis, haemarthrosis, gout and pseudogout.
- Joints with acute gout show the presence of negatively birefringent crystals on analysis with polarized light.
- Pseudogout shows the presence of positively birefringent crystals.
- Gout typically occurs in the large toe joint; also look for evidence of gouty tophi in the helix of the ear and on the fingers.
- Osteoarthritis is more likely in those over the age of 40, often affecting weight-bearing joints.
- In the clinical exam ensure that you identify carefully the site of maximal tenderness. The examiners may be offering you a case of bursitis. In this case the tenderness will be localized and the joint will show a full range of movement.

Rheumatology

Psoriatic arthritis

Most **S**uffer **R**heumatoid **O**r **D**IP

Mutilans
Sacroiliitis
Rheumatoid-like
Oligoarthritis
Distal interphalangeal (DIP) joint

Topic facts

The five types of psoriatic arthritis are summarized above.

- Rheumatoid-like psoriatic arthritis is the most common form of psoriatic arthropathy, followed by oligoarthritis, DIP joint, sacroiliitis and mutilans.
- It is important on examination of joint disease patients to look thoroughly for evidence of psoriasis. Patients may have extensive joint involvement with minimal skin involvement.
- Do not be caught out in patients with rheumatoid-like psoriatic arthritis. You can be sure the diagnosis is rheumatoid arthritis only if rheumatoid nodules are present (typically found on the extensor surface at the elbows).
- Skin changes are typically found on the extensor surfaces, but look especially in the hairline, ears and umbilicus.
- Do not forget to look for skin and joint changes in the legs and feet. These may be the only sites of involvement.
- Nail changes associated with psoriasis:
  - pitting
  - hyperkeratosis
  - onycholysis (separation of the nail plate from underlying attachment to the nail-bed).
- Treatment includes steroid joint injections and immunosuppressants such as methotrexate.

Raynaud's phenomenon

Icy **C**old **H**ands
   Idiopathic (young women)
   Connective tissue disease
   Hand tools that vibrate

Topic facts

Raynaud's phenomenon is the result of peripheral vasoconstriction, resulting in characteristic changes of skin colour in the hands. This mnemonic lists the more common causes of Raynaud's phenomenon.

- The order of colour change is white, blue, red.
- The white pallor is the result of poor blood supply to the affected region during vasoconstriction. The blue colour is caused by cyanosis and the red colour change occurs on vasodilatation as a result of hyperaemia.
- There are many common causes of Raynaud's phenomenon; the most common are listed in the mnemonic.
- Idiopathic Raynaud's phenomenon is present from a young age and is more commonly found in females. It is an independent phenomenon not associated with other diseases. Cold exposure is the most common stimulus.
- Secondary Raynaud's phenomenon presents at a later age (typically older than 30 years) and is associated with the connective tissue diseases (see page 162) and use of vibrating hand tools.
- Systemic sclerosis is the most common connective tissue disease associated with Raynaud's phenomenon.
- Rarer causes of secondary Raynaud's phenomenon include haematological malignancies (myeloma, leukaemia, polycythaemia), endocrine disorders (hypothyroid, phaeochromocytoma, carcinoid) and neurological disorders (cervical spondylosis, syringomyelia, multiple sclerosis).

Rheumatology

Reiter's syndrome
PEA
Penis (urethritis)
Eyes (conjunctivitis)
Arthritis

Topic facts
Reiter's syndrome comprises the triad of reactive arthritis, conjunctivitis and urethritis, as summarized in this mnemonic.

- Reiter's syndrome is more common in men, and presents from the late teens to the early 40s.
- This syndrome is associated with HLA-B27 positivity (HLA-B27 expression is associated with the seronegative spondyloarthropathies such as ankylosing spondylitis).
- *Chlamydia* sp. is the most common causative organism.
- Other causes include *Shigella*, *Salmonella* and *Mycoplasma* spp.
- Complications of Reiter's syndrome include:
  - **keratoderma blenorrhagica**: a brownish-red maculopapular rash found on the palms and soles with some vesicopustules
  - **circinate balanitis**: painless ulcers on the glans of the penis in up to a quarter of affected people
  - **uveitis**.
- Patients complain of fever, malaise, myalgia and joint stiffness 1–3 weeks after an episode of urethritis, cervicitis or diarrhoea.
- Prognosis is good with resolution in the majority (though recurrence occurs in a minority).
- Treatment of the arthritis is symptomatic with analgesia. Urethritis and conjunctivitis require antibiotic therapy.

Rheumatology

Rheumatoid arthritis

Rheumatoid **A**rthritis **V**ery **O**ften **C**auses **P**ulmonary **F**ibrosis

Rheumatoid nodules

Anaemia

Vasculitis

Osteoporosis

Carpal tunnel syndrome

Pleurisy/**P**yoderma gangrenosum/**P**ericarditis

Fibrosis (lung)/**F**elty's syndrome

A disease of thirds

A third have cervical spine disease

A third have extra-articular involvement

A third have eye involvement

Topic facts

The first memory aid lists the complications associated with rheumatoid arthritis. The second summarizes the frequency of common complications.

- Clinical features:
  - swan-neck deformity
  - Boutonnière's deformity
  - Z thumb
  - wasting of the small muscles of the hand
  - ulnar deviation
  - synovitis particularly of the MCP (metacarpophalangeal) joints.
- Complications not listed in the mnemonic include:
  - scleritis
  - ischaemic heart disease
  - episcleritis
  - Cushing's syndrome (from steroid use).
- Felty's syndrome is the triad of splenomegaly, leukopenia and lymphadenopathy.

Rheumatoid arthritis (continued)

Might **G**ive **S**ome **P**enicillamine
  Methotrexate
  Gold
  Sulfasalazine
  Penicillamine

Topic facts

The treatment options used in rheumatoid arthritis are summarized here.

- First-line treatment is now with disease-modifying anti-rheumatoid drugs (DMARDs).
- DMARDs are superior to non-steroidal anti-inflammatory drugs (NSAIDs) without being more toxic in the long term.
- Delayed introduction of DMARDs is associated with a worse outcome.
- Methotrexate is the first-line treatment. It is usually given as a weekly dose. Patients are given folic acid supplements. Side-effects include hepatic fibrosis, bone marrow suppression and pneumonitis. Patients require monitoring of full blood count and liver function while on treatment.
- Sulfasalazine is often used as second-line treatment,
- Gold is now less commonly used and has a poor side-effect profile (including proteinuria, cytopenia and diarrhoea).
- Steroids may be required during episodes of acute arthritis.
- Patients who fail to respond to DMARD therapy may benefit from anti-tumour necrosis factor α (anti-TNF-α).
- Anti-TNF-α drugs such as the monoclonal antibody infliximab may provide significant improvement, although the long-term side-effect profile is as yet unclear.
- NSAIDs have a role in providing symptomatic relief.

Seronegative arthritis

Arthritic **P**ain **E**xcluding **R**heumatoid

   Ankylosing spondylitis

   Psoriatic arthritis

   Enteropathic arthritis

   Reiter's syndrome (reactive arthritis)

Topic facts

The disorders that make up the seronegative arthritis group are summarized in this mnemonic.

- The seronegative arthritides are associated with HLA-B27 (seronegative refers to the absence of rheumatoid factor).
- Enteropathic arthritis encompasses the seronegative arthritis associated with ulcerative colitis and Crohn's disease.
- The activity of the bowel disease is often reflected in the degree of joint involvement.
- Five per cent of patients with inflammatory bowel disease develop ankylosing spondylitis.
- The most common seronegative arthropathy is ankylosing spondylitis (see page 159).
- Common clinical features:
  - dactylitis (sausage-shaped swelling of the digits)
  - enthesitis (inflammation and pain at the point where the tendon inserts into the bone)
  - sacroiliitis (inflammation of the sacroiliac joints).
- Ankylosing spondylitis (see page 159) presents in young to middle-aged adults, commonly male, with a history of morning stiffness and back pain. Patients develop the characteristic question mark posture.
- Calcification of the interspinous ligaments leads to the characteristic bamboo appearance on a radiograph.

Rheumatology

Vasculitis
CRAP WIGS

Churg–Strauss syndrome (asthma + eosinophilia)

Rheumatoid arthritis (joint changes)

Antiphospholipid syndrome (clots, miscarriages, livedo reticularis)

Polyarteritis nodosa (weight loss, neuropathy, livedo reticularis)

Wegener's granulomatosis (3 Rs – rhinitis, respiratory and renal involvement)

Infection (hepatitis B, C, *Staphylococcus aureus*) Infective endocarditis

Giant cell arteritis (jaw claudication, pain on combing hair, association with PMR polymyalgia rheumatica [PMR])

SLE (typical photosensitive rash, associated arthritis)

(Also consider Kawasaki's disease, Takayasu's arteritis and Henoch–Schönlein purpura.)

Topic facts

The more common vasculitic diseases are given here with their associated findings in brackets.

- The vasculitides are a group of disorders that result in inflammation of the blood vessels.
- The common clinical findings are fever, malaise, weight loss and a vasculitic rash (palpable purpura).
- Look in the history and/or examination for the key associated findings to identify the correct type.
- Categorize vasculitis by vessel size:
  - large:
    - giant cell
    - Takayasu's arteritis
  - medium:
    - polyarteritis nodosa
    - Kawasaki's disease:
  - small
    - the rest.

Infectious diseases

- AIDS + CD4 count
- Antibiotics with anaerobic activity
- Herpes zoster
- Lymphadenopathy (generalized)
- Malignant external otitis
- Meningitis
- Prion diseases
- Secondary syphilis
- Vaccines

AIDS + CD4 count

Sexually Transmitted Particles Take CD4 Titres

CD4 count (cells/mm³)	Infection risk
300	**S**yphilis
	Tuberculosis (**T**B)
200	Pneumocystis carinii pneumonia (**P**CP)
	Toxoplasma sp.
100	Cytomegalovirus reticutus (**C**MV)
	Tuberculosis atypical (**T**B)

Topic facts

This topic summarizes the opportunistic infections to which individuals are at risk, dependent on their CD4 count.

- *Toxoplasma* sp. is one of the most common HIV-related opportunistic infectious organisms.
- AIDS-defining conditions:
  - PCP
  - TB
  - cryptosporidiasis
  - CMV retinitis
  - oral hairy leucoplakia
- When to start treatment
  - CD4 <500
  - symptomatic patients
  - rapidly dropping CD4 count
  - viral load >10 000 copies
- Treatment is with HAART (highly active antiretroviral therapy).
- Starting regimen is two NRTIs (nucleoside reverse transcriptase inhibitors) and a PI (protease inhibitor).

Antibiotics with anaerobic activity

Metronidazole **C**omes **T**op

  Metronidazole

  Clindamycin/**C**hloramphenicol/**C**ephalosporins

  Tetracycline

Topic facts

The antibiotics that are active against anaerobes are summarized here.

Antibiotic groups

- Anti-bacterial DNA antibiotics:
    - quinolones (ciprofloxacin, levofloxacin)
    - sulphonamides (sulfadiazine)
    - trimethoprim
    - nitroimidazoles (metronidazole).
- Anti-bacterial cell wall antibiotics:
    - penicillins (phenoxymethylpenicillin, amoxicillin, flucloxacillin)
    - cephalosporins (cefuroxime, cefotaxime)
    - vancomycin
    - β-lactams (meropenem).
- Bacterial protein synthesis inhibitors:
    - macrolides (erythromycin, clarithromycin)
    - aminoglycosides (gentamicin)
    - tetracyclines.
- The quinolones prevent replication by the inhibition of DNA gyrase. (This enzyme is necessary to allow the bacterial DNA to supercoil and fit inside the small bacterial nucleus. Eukaryotic cells in humans are larger so the DNA does not supercoil.)
- Bactericidal antibiotics kill bacteria; bacteriostatic ones prevent replication.

Infectious diseases

Herpes zoster

PVC Scar
   Papule
   Vesicle
   Crusting
   Scar

Topic facts

The order of progression of lesions found in secondary herpes zoster infection is given in the mnemonic.

- Primary herpes zoster infection presents as chickenpox, typically in childhood.
- If primary infection occurs in adulthood, the course may be more severe.
- Secondary infection presents as shingles with the characteristic dermatomal distribution and herpetiform rash.
- Clusters are seen containing lesions at the different stages of development. The order of lesion formation is listed in the mnemonic.
- Most patients with shingles are aged >50 years.
- Immunosuppressed patients are at higher risk of infection:
  - elderly people
  - those on immunosuppressive treatment
  - those with acquired immunodeficiency secondary to malignancy or infection.
- Complications include post-herpetic neuralgia (which may respond to amitriptyline, carbamazepine, gabapentin, pregabalin or topical capsaicin), ophthalmic zoster and Ramsay Hunt syndrome.
- Ramsay Hunt syndrome occurs as a result of herpes zoster of the geniculate ganglion (part of cranial nerve VII). There is weakness of facial muscles and vesicles are seen in the ear canal.

Lymphadenopathy (generalized)

Tender **S**wollen **G**lands **A**re **C**ommon

*T*oxoplasma sp.

Syphilis

Glandular fever (Epstein–Barr virus)

AIDS

Cytomegalovirus

Topic facts

The more common infective causes of generalized lymphadenopathy are summarized here.

- Generalized tender lymphadenopathy with a history of fever is suggestive of an infective cause.
- Infective glands are typically tender to palpation and mobile.
- Persistent enlargement of lymph nodes is suggestive of lymphoma or leukaemia (see pages 9–11).
- If the patient is acutely unwell or if lymphadenopathy is persistent, further investigation is warranted.
- Investigations:
  - full blood count (FBC):
    high white cell counts in infection or haematological malignancy
  - blood film:
    smear cells in chronic lymphatic leukaemia (fragile lymphocytes that burst open on the microscopy slide)
  - lymph node biopsy:
    the most diagnostically useful test but invasive
  - fine-needle aspiration:
    less invasive but has a low diagnostic yield
  - bone marrow biopsy:
    useful in the leukaemias.

Infectious diseases

Malignant external otitis

*Pseudomonas **Ear**-ruginosa*

Topic facts

Pseudomonas aeruginosa is a Gram-negative organism and an important cause of nosocomial (hospital-acquired) infection. It is the causative organism of malignant external otitis.

- Malignant external otitis is usually preceded by a normal external otitis (pain and ear discharge), which then fails to respond to a course of antibiotics.
- Invasive infection occurs when there is extension into the soft tissue and underlying temporal bone. If infection is not controlled it may extend to the central nervous system (CNS).
- Clinical features indicating development of invasive infection:
  - worsening of pain despite antibiotic course
  - purulent discharge.
- In some cases cranial nerve palsies develop.
- The high mortality rate associated with this condition has resulted in the usage of the term 'malignant'.
- Invasive infection is more common in patients with poorly controlled diabetes mellitus.
- Investigation:
  - full blood count (FBC)
  - swabs of discharge
  - imaging with CT or MRI if extension into the temporal bone or abscess is suspected.
- Treatment of infection requires two antibiotics for 4–8 weeks ± surgery.
- Ceftazidime is the treatment of choice in those with extension into the CNS.
- *P. aeruginosa* is a common organism of infection in immunocompromised individuals.

Meningitis
Every **L**ittle **B**aby
Must **H**ave **P**rotection (to)
Stop **M**eningitis

Babies
E. coli
Listeria sp.
Beta-haemolytic streptococci

Kids
Meningococcal (*Neisseria meningitidis*)
Haemophilus influenzae
Pneumococci (*Streptococcus pneumoniae*)

Adults
S. pneumoniae
Meningococcal (*N. meningitidis*)

Topic facts
The common causative organisms of meningitis are summarized here categorized by age group.

- Causative agents for meningitis vary with age group.
- If meningitis is suspected, blood cultures should be taken and empirical treatment commenced followed by lumbar puncture.
- Empirical treatment for adults with suspected bacterial meningitis is cefotaxime + benzylpenicillin.
- The most common causes of meningitis worldwide are *S. pneumoniae*, *N. meningitidis* and *H. influenzae*.
- Gram stain helps differentiate these three causes. If shown a slide, Gram positive stains purple and Gram negative stains pink. *S. pneumoniae* is Gram positive, and both *N. meningitidis* and *H. influenzae* are Gram negative.

Infectious diseases

Prion diseases
F*CK
>**F**atal familial insomnia
>**C**reutzfeldt–Jakob disease (CJD)
>**K**uru

Topic facts
Prion diseases are a group of disorders that result in neurological damage and eventually death. The common prion diseases are summarized here.

- Prions are thought to be a protein-only particle, which mimics normal cell surface proteins.
- Many prion diseases are also TSEs – transmissible spongiform encephalopathies.
- Typically there is a long period of time between exposure and onset of symptoms.
- Once symptoms develop the course of deterioration is usually rapid (mean survival in CJD is 8 months).
- Prions are thought to infect cells by converting normal cell surface proteins to prion proteins on coming into contact with them.
- CJD presents with a rapid-onset dementia and myoclonus.
- New variant CJD has a slower course, presenting with memory impairment and irritability, followed by loss of coordination, hyperreflexia and myoclonus. Mean survival is 16 months.
- An interesting aside is that kuru was once spread through tribes involved with cannibalism in New Guinea (which involved consumption of brain tissue).
- Prion diseases in animals include scrapie in sheep and bovine spongiform encephalopathy (BSE) in cattle.

Prusiner SB. Novel proteinaceous infectious particles cause scrapie. *Science* 1982;**216**: 136–44.

Secondary syphilis

Syphilis **T**wo – **P**ink **L**ooking **M**acules

Syphilis
Tinea versicolor
Pityriasis rosea
Lichen planus
Mononucleosis

Topic facts

The differential diagnosis for the macular appearance of secondary syphilis is shown above.

- Secondary syphilis typically presents 1–3 months after the onset of the initial lesion (genital chancre).
- The clinical appearance is of reddish-brown macules, up to 0.5 cm in diameter on the palms and soles.
- As the rash progresses, macules, papules and pustules may be found on the trunk and face.
- Mucosal patches may develop orally or genitally and are a source of transmission. (Transmission occurs mainly through unprotected sexual intercourse.)
- Patients may complain of malaise, loss of appetite, fever and headache.
- Investigations:
  - syphilis serology (Venereal Disease Research Laboratory [VDRL] – 80 per cent sensitivity in primary syphilis and 99 per cent in secondary but poor specificity; the fluorescent treponemal antibody absorption test [FTA-Abs] is used to confirm a positive VDRL result)
  - darkfield microscopy.
- Treatment is with penicillins or doxycycline.
- There are four syphilitic stages: primary, secondary, latent and tertiary syphilis.
- Primary lesions occur approximately 3 weeks after infection at the site of transmission. They are raised, firm papules that may ulcerate and are typically painless.

Infectious diseases

Vaccines (live)
MMR BOY
Measles
Mumps
Rubella
BCG
Oral polio
Yellow fever

Topic facts
The live vaccines are summarized above.

- There are four main types of vaccine available: live attenuated, killed organism, preformed antibody and subunit vaccines.
- Live attenuated vaccines are made from strains of live virus with low virulence (common examples are listed in the mnemonic).
- Killed organism vaccines are inactivated using heat or chemicals and produce a lesser immune response. However, they are safe and commonly given to elderly and immunocompromised people, e.g. the yearly flu vaccines.
- Preformed antibody vaccines are given to acutely infected individuals, to help bind antigen and aid clearance, e.g. rabies antibody vaccine.
- Subunit vaccines are made from parts of the virus that stimulate a beneficial immune response, e.g. hepatitis B subunit vaccine.
- The MMR triple vaccine contains three live attenuated viruses and is given to children aged 2–15 months and a booster at 3 years. BCG (bacille Calmette–Guérin) is given at birth to high-risk babies: it is no longer given routinely (Don 2005 Voccinetion program).
- Live vaccines are contraindicated in immunocompromised individuals where even attenuated strains may lead to full-blown infection.

Dermatology

- Erythema nodosum
- Henoch–Schönlein purpura
- Koebner's phenomenon
- Livedo reticularis
- Malignant melanoma
- Pellagra
- Peutz–Jeghers syndrome
- Photosensitive skin reactions
- Purpura

Erythema nodosum
SPLIT

Sarcoid
Streptococcal infection
Sjögren's syndrome
SLE (systemic lupus erythematosus)
Sulphonamides

Pregnancy
Penicillin
Pill (oral contraceptive pill)
Psittacosis

Leprosy
Lymphogranuloma venerum

Inflammatory bowel disease (IBD)

Tuberculosis (TB)

Topic facts

The more common causes of erythema nodosum are summarized here.

- Erythema nodosum (EN) presents as raised tender red lesions over the shins (if very tense the skin may appear about to *split*).
- Streptococcal infection is the most common cause of erythema nodosum, followed by sarcoid-related and IBD-related EN.
- IBD-related EN is improved by effective control of the inflammatory bowel disease.
- Patients with Löfgren's syndrome (see page 142) have a better prognosis than other sarcoid patients with lung involvement (with regard to resolution of pulmonary fibrosis).

Henoch–Schönlein purpura
You see HSP in a rash-ridden kiddy

Topic facts

- Henoch–Schönlein purpura (HSP) is a small-vessel vasculitis and the most common childhood vasculitis. The presentation is summarized in this memory aid.
- Clinical findings are of a purpuric rash covering the lower limbs and buttocks. The rash is pruritic and most prominent over the extensor surfaces.
- Most cases are in children and young adults.
- Additional features include:
  - arthralgia (occurs in the majority)
  - colicky abdominal pain
  - diarrhoea (± blood)
  - renal involvement (haematuria and proteinuria on dipstick).
- Investigation: primarily a clinical diagnosis, skin biopsy reveals a leukocytoclastic vasculitis with IgA deposition.
- Most patients have a full recovery without medical intervention.
- A minority go on to develop glomerulonephritis and nephritic or nephrotic syndrome, for which corticosteroid treatment is required.
- In HSP there is an IgA-dominant deposition and it is associated with Berger's disease – IgA nephropathy.
- Complications of HSP:
  - gastrointestinal bleeding
  - gastrointestinal perforation
  - intussusception
  - renal failure.

Koebner's phenomenon

Warts **M**ake **A** **P**retty **L**ine
> **W**arts
> **M**olluscum contagiosum
> **A**utoimmune (vitiligo)
> **P**soriasis/**P**emphigus
> **L**ichen planus

Topic facts

The topic lists common conditions that koebnerize.

- Koebner's phenomenon is the formation of new skin lesions on areas of apparently normal skin after trauma (e.g. a scratch leading to the formation of a line of warts over the affected area).
- A brief summary of the appearance and key information of the conditions is given below:
  - **molluscum contagiosum** has a pearly white appearance and umbilicated centre (it is caused by a pox virus and resolves spontaneously within 18 months; lesions are contagious and immunosuppressed adults may develop these in large numbers)
  - **vitiligo** presents as an area of hypopigmented skin; it may be a marker of organ-specific autoimmune disease (see page 124)
  - **psoriasis** presents with characteristic silver plaques on a red base; the hairline is often involved; koebnerization is common
  - **pemphigus** presents with superficial fragile bullae (as opposed to the tense bullae of pemphigoid)
  - **lichen planus** is a violaceous, pruritic, raised lesion covered by a lacy white streaking (Wickham's striae); check the buccal mucosa where striae are more prominent.

Dermatology

Livedo reticularis

A Horrible **V**asculitis **C**ase

    Antiphospholipid

    Hyperviscosity

    Vasculitides

    Cholesterol emboli/**C**ryoglobulinaemia

Topic facts

Livedo reticularis is a dermatological phenomenon with a characteristic marbled appearance of violaceous streaks and central pallor. The causes of livedo are summarized above.

- Livedo reticularis can occur independently or in association with the conditions listed above.
- Antiphospholipid syndrome results from circulating antibodies (IgG and IgM) against phospholipids. It is associated with systemic lupus and other autoimmune diseases.
  - associated findings in antiphospholipid syndrome:
    - arterial and venous clots
    - recurrent abortions
    - pulmonary hypertension
    - transient ischaemic attack (TIA)/stroke
    - chorea
    - migraine
    - thrombocytopenia
  - investigation (AS): anticardiolipin antibody, prolongation of activated partial thromboplastin time (APTT) on addition of normal plasma as a result of the lupus anticoagulant effect.
  - management (AS): anticoagulation.
- Hyperviscosity states include paraproteinaemias, myeloma, Waldenström's macroglobulinaemia and polycythaemia rubra vera.
- Cholesterol emboli can occur as a complication of thrombolysis, anticoagulation and angiography.

Malignant melanoma
ABCDE
Asymmetry
Border irregularity
Colour variation
Diameter >6 mm
Evolving lesions

Topic facts
This mnemonic is a memory aid to the early diagnosis of malignant melanoma.

- Malignant melanoma is a malignant tumour of the melanocytes associated with sun exposure and is more common in non-pigmented skin. (Albinos are particularly predisposed to this condition.)
- A small number of cases are autosomal dominant inherited and may develop multiple malignancies.
- Individuals with atypical mole syndrome have abnormally high numbers of moles and are at increased risk of developing malignant melanoma.
- The most commonly affected sites are the leg and trunk (although lesions of the head and neck are also common).
- Lesions are most commonly identified in the early 60s.
- Malignant melanoma has two growth phases: radial and vertical. Vertical growth is associated with a poor prognosis.
- Most malignant melanomas are >10 mm in diameter.
- 'Evolving lesions' refers to changes in size, shape, symptoms (itching, tenderness) or surface (especially bleeding and colour change).

Rigel DS, Friedman RJ, Kopf AW, Polsky D. ABCDE an evolving concept in the early detection of melanoma. *Arch Dermatol* 2005;**141**:1032–4.

Pellagra
5 Ds
Dermatitis

Dementia

Diarrhoea

Death

Due to niacin deficiency

Topic facts
The 5 Ds are a well-known mnemonic summarizing the findings associated with pellagra.

- Pellagra is the result of niacin (Vitamin B_3) deficiency.
- Niacin deficiency may be a consequence of malabsorption, carcinoid syndrome, isoniazid therapy or alcohol dependence.
- Isoniazid is a pyridoxine antagonist (an important step in the pathway producing nicotinic acid). Pyridoxine supplementation prevents this complication.
- Carcinoid syndrome also interrupts the pathway, through consumption of precursors.
- Dermatitis most commonly affects the dorsal aspect of the hands, face, neck, arms and feet.
- The neck may be particularly affected (Casal necklace).
- Lesions are initially red and painful and fade to a brown–red colour.
- Psychiatric involvement may vary from irritability and poor concentration through to memory loss, stupor and coma.
- Other findings in pellagra:
  - stomatitis
  - ataxia
  - fits
  - depression
  - increased tone.

Dermatology

Peutz–Jeghers syndrome
PPP

Peutz–Jeghers syndrome
Pigmentation
Polyps

Topic facts
Peutz–Jegher syndrome is an autosomal dominant inherited disorder.
- The following are the clinical features of Peutz–Jeghers syndrome:
  - pigmented macules around the mouth (there may also be pigmentation of the buccal mucosa)
  - hamartomatous polyps in the gastrointestinal tract, especially in the jejunum.
- Complications:
  - recurrent abdominal pain
  - intestinal obstruction
  - intussusception
  - gastrointestinal bleeding
  - iron deficiency anaemia.
- Peutz–Jeghers syndrome is associated with cancer of the ovary, lung, breast and pancreas.
- Treatment is symptomatic. Polypectomy may be required if symptoms are severe.
- See memory aid for auto somal dominout conditions (page 209).

Photosensitive skin reaction
DIM

Drugs **(PANTS)**
- **P**henothiazines
- **A**miodarone
- **N**on-steroidal anti-inflammatory drugs (NSAIDs)
- **T**hiazides, **T**etracyclines
- **S**ulphonamides

Immune
- Systemic lupus erythematosus (SLE)
- Dermatomyositis
- Albinism

Metabolic
- Porphyrias (cutanea tarda, erythropoietic)
- Pellagra (5 Ds)

Topic facts
Photosensitive skin reactions are seen best on areas of exposed skin such as the forehead, pinna of the ears and base of the neck. The causes are categorized by this mnemonic into drug, immune and metabolic photosensitivity.
- Acute intermittent porphyria is *not* associated with a photosensitive rash.
- Use of PUVA (psoralen and UV A) treatment for psoriatic patients while on potentially photosensitizing treatment (eg a thiazide diuretic) is a potential hazard.
- Cutanea tarda results from deficiency of uroporphyrinogen decarboxylase.
- Treatment of photosensitive patients includes use of alternative drugs, avoidance of sun exposure and use of anti-UV skin creams on exposed areas.

Dermatology

Purpura
Capillary/Platelet/Coagulation

Capillary

Inherited
- Collagen diseases (see pg 161)
- Hereditary haemorrhagic telangiectasia

Acquired
- Severe infection
- Purpuras (senile, steroid, Henoch–Schönlein)

Platelet
- Idiopathic thrombocytopenic purpura (young women ± splenomegaly)
- Marrow infiltration (secondaries, leukaemia)
- Marrow aplasia (drugs, viral)

Coagulation
- Anticoagulant treatment
- Haemophilia A or B
- Von Willebrand's disease

Topic facts

The common causes of purpura (bruising) are summarized here. This mnemonic is identical to that of bleeding disorders (see page 5) because the presence of purpura is a cardinal sign of a bleeding disorder.

- Platelet abnormalities are suggested by petechial bleeding (pinpoint purpura).
- Steroid treatment and unexplained 'senile purpura' are the most common causes of purpura seen by doctors.
- Coagulation disorders are also common, especially iatrogenic cases from the treatment of deep vein thrombosis, atrial fibrillation, pulmonary embolus and other thrombotic states.

Part 1 sciences: biochemistry and metabolism

- Acute phase reactants
- Cyclic AMP + G protein disease
- Drugs affected by cytochrome P450 inhibition/induction
- Enzyme inducers and inhibitors
- Hypercalcaemia
- Hyperlipidaemia
- Hypernatraemia
- Hyperpyrexia
- Hyperuricaemia
- Hypocalcaemia
- Hypokalaemia
- Metabolic acidosis
- Metabolic alkalosis
- Slow acetylators
- Syndrome of inappropriate ADH secretion
- Tetany

Acute phase reactants

Acute **I**nflammatory **C**omponents

Alpha$_1$-antitrypsin
Alpha-glycoprotein
Alpha-macroglobulin
Amyloid

Iron (ferritin)

Complement
C-reactive protein (CRP)
Caeruloplasmin

Topic facts

This topic covers the components that form part of the acute inflammatory response.

- The acute phase reactants are plasma proteins that are produced during the acute phase response.
- The acute phase response occurs when there is tissue damage such as inflammation, infection, ischaemic damage or trauma.
- Other important acute phase reactants include fibrinogen and haptoglobin.
- D-dimer, a measure of fibrin degradation products, is used to evaluate the presence of clot in the body for patients with suspected pulmonary embolus or deep vein thrombosis. As fibrinogen is raised by the acute phase reaction, D-dimer may also be elevated, despite the absence of clot.
- Similarly, ferritin levels and α_1-antitrypsin levels are elevated and testing for these during an acute phase response may lead to inaccurate results.
- CRP is used as a measure of the acute phase response in order to monitor disease progress or response to treatment, e.g. in systemic infection.

Cyclic AMP + G protein disease
G-CAMP
G-protein linked disease
Cholera
Acromegaly
McCune–Albright syndrome
Pseudohypoparathyroidism

Topic facts
G proteins are cell surface receptors that use cyclic AMP (cAMP) as an intracellular messenger. (G proteins can use other second messengers but cAMP is the most common.) Common G-protein-linked diseases are summarized above.
- There are two types: stimulatory leading to higher levels of intracellular cAMP and inhibitory leading to lower levels.
- Most hormones are stimulatory (somatostatin is the exception).
- Cholera toxin binds to a G protein causing permanent activation, leading to the secretory diarrhoea that occurs.
- Acromegaly is associated with an activating somatic mutation of G proteins, leading to permanently 'switched-on' pituitary cells causing excessive growth hormone secretion.
- McCune–Albright syndrome is an activating G-protein mutation leading to hyperfunction of endocrine glands. Features include precocious puberty.
- Pseudohypoparathyroidism is the result of an inactivating G-protein mutation that leads to resistance to hormones that act via cAMP, including parathyroid hormone thyroid-stimulating hormone (TSH) and gonadotrophins.

Drugs affected by cytochrome P450 inhibition/induction

Warfarin **TOP**

Warfarin
Theophylline
Oral contraceptive pill
Phenytoin

Topic facts

Common drugs metabolized by the enzyme cytochrome P450 system are listed in this topic.

- The cytochrome P450 enzyme system is an important liver-based group of 40–50 enzymes, responsible for the clearance of many endogenous waste products and some drugs.
- Both drugs and diet can induce or inhibit the cytochrome P450 system; the drugs that affect the rate of cytochrome P450 metabolism are discussed on page 195.
- Cauliflower and cabbage are inducers and grapefruit juice is an inhibitor of cytochrome P450.
- Enzyme induction can lead to subtherapeutic drug levels as a result of increased clearance of drug.
- Conversely, enzyme inhibition can lead to a build-up to toxic drug levels in the plasma as a result of a failure to clear the drug.
- To avoid inadequate or excessive treatment doses, it is important to counsel patients taking drugs affected by enzyme induction or inhibition, and to inform any doctors or pharmacists of their medication before accepting changes in their treatment.
- In particular, women of childbearing age are at risk of pregnancy if taking the oral contraceptive and prescribed an enzyme-inducing agent, e.g. rifampicin. Patients should be advised to use alternative methods of contraception.
- Patients on warfarin therapy require close monitoring until levels become stabilized on a regular treatment regimen.

Enzyme inducers and inhibitors

Enzyme inducers
SCRAP

Sulphonamides
Carbamazepine
Rifampicin
Alcohol (chronic usage)
Phenytoin

Enzyme inhibitors
ICE DOVE

Isoniazid
Cimetidine/**C**iprofloxacin
Erythromycin

Disulfiram
Omeprazole
Valproate (sodium)
Ethanol (acute intoxication)

Topic facts
The enzyme-inducing and -inhibiting drugs are summarized in the two memory aids above.
- Enzyme-inducing drugs lead to activation of the cytochrome P450 enzyme system in the liver.
- The cytochrome P450 system is important in metabolizing active drugs into inactive states.
- Increased drug metabolism may lead to less than therapeutic drug levels.
- Inhibited metabolism may lead to toxic drug levels.
- Important drugs metabolized by the cytochrome P450 enzymes are discussed on page 194.

Hypercalcaemia (>3.5 mmol/L)

Bony **M**ets **P**roduce **V**ery **B**ig **C**alcium

Bone disease (metastasis)

Milk alkali syndrome/**M**yeloma

Parathyroid (primary, parathyroid hormone-related peptide or PTHrp)

Vitamin D excess

Benign familial hypocalciuric hypercalcaemia

Chronic renal failure, i.e. tertiary hyperparathyroidism

Topic facts

Causes of severe hypercalcaemia (calcium level > 3.5 mmol/L) are given in this memory aid.

- Primary hyperparathyroidism is the most common cause of hypercalcaemia followed by cancer-related hypercalcaemia.
- Parathyroid hormone (PTH) acts on two main targets to increase plasma calcium concentration. In the kidneys it promotes calcium absorption and vitamin D activation (it also promotes phosphate excretion) and in bone it stimulates osteoclasts to release calcium and phosphate.
- Cancer-related hypercalaemia may be from bony metastasis or PTHrp production.
- PTHrp is able to stimulate the normal PTH receptors in the kidney and bones. Cancers that release PTHrp include renal adenocarcinoma, squamous cell lung cancer and some ovarian tumours.
- Lower levels of hypercalcaemia are associated with endocrine disease such as hyperthyroidism, Addison's disease, acromegaly and phaeochromocytoma.
- Long-term immobility can also lead to hypercalcaemia.
- Hypercalcaemia is a medical emergency. Calcium levels >3.7 mmol/L can be fatal. Treatment involves rehydration and bisphosphonates.

Hyperlipidaemia

Eating **T**reats **P**roduces **F**atties

    Eruptive xanthoma: type 1

    Tendon xanthoma: type 2a

    Palmar xanthoma: type 3

    Fatty-looking blood: type 4

Topic facts

The key clinical findings associated with the familial hyperlipidaemias, in order of type, are summarized in this topic.

- The primary hyperlipidaemias are a group of disorders classified by the lipid component that is elevated:
  - type 1 (elevated chylomicrons)
  - type 2a (elevated low-density lipoprotein or LDL)
  - type 3 (elevated intermediate-density lipoprotein or IDL)
  - type 4 (elevated very-low-density lipoprotein or VLDL).
- Type 1 is an autosomal recessive condition caused by elevated triglyceride levels stored in chylomicrons. It is the result of apo-CII or lipoprotein lipase deficiency. The clinical finding is eruptive xanthoma, and the complication pancreatitis.
- Type 2a (familial hypercholesterolaemia) is an autosomal dominant disorder of elevated cholesterol (LDL). It is the result of a deficiency of LDL receptors. The complication is atherosclerotic disease. Prognosis is poor if left untreated (death in early 20s).
- Type 3 hyperlipidaemia is a rare hyperlipidaemia caused by elevated IDL (chylomicron remnant particles). It is the result of a defect of apolipoprotein E. Patients present with atherosclerotic disease and palmar xanthoma.
- Type 4 (familial hypertriglyceridaemia) is an autosomal dominant inherited condition caused by elevated VLDL (triglyceride). Blood is a creamy-white colour as a result of high levels of lipid.
- Statins are the mainstay of lipid reduction therapy.

Hypernatraemia

Over-**D**ehydration
  Osmotic diuresis
  Dehydration/**D**iabetes insipidus

Topic facts

Common causes of hypernatraemia are given above.

- Hypernatraemia is the result of excess water loss relative to sodium.
- Dehydration is the most common cause and may be the result of poor intake, particularly in elderly and young people who may not be able to meet their water needs. Thirst sensation is not as acute in elderly people and may also be a contributory factor.
- Other factors include losses from the skin and lungs, particularly in hot environments or after burn injuries or diarrhoea.
- Osmotic diuresis should be considered in those with type 2 diabetes. Hypernatraemia commonly occurs in Hyper Osmolar Non Ketotic diabetic syndrome (HONK).
- Diabetes insipidus of pituitary origin leads to hypernatraemia as a result of failure to produce antidiuretic hormone (ADH).
- Polyuria and polydipsia are present.
- Failure to replace fluids lost results in hypernatraemia and a fluid-depleted state.
- Hypernatraemia requires careful management because rapid correction can be fatal if cerebral oedema ensues.
- In cases with sodium levels >170 mmol/L, physiological or 0.9 per cent saline should be used to enable a gradual correction of the hypernatraemia.
- Physiological (or normal) saline solution is isotonic with normal serum plasma but hypotonic compared with that of a hypernatraemic patient; it thus lowers sodium levels gradually, unlike 5 per cent dextrose which may cause a rapid and dangerous correction.

Hyperpyrexia

(hot) **PANTS**

Prostaglandins
Amphetamine
Neuroleptic malignant syndrome
Thyroid storm
Septicaemia

Topic facts

Hyperpyrexia is defined as a core temperature >41°C; the differential is given in this topic.

- Management of hyperpyrexia includes removal of any precipitating factors (drug, infection), cooling with sponging, paracetamol and dantrolene. Fits may be precipitated by hyperpyrexia and should be managed with lorazepam.
- Amphetamine abuse (e.g. ecstasy – MDMA) is suggested by the presence of dilated pupils, tachycardia, hypertension and excessive sweating.
- Neuroleptic malignant syndrome is an idiosyncratic reaction to a neuroleptic drug, e.g. haloperidol or metoclopramide. Serum creatinine kinase levels are high.
- Thyroid storm is a medical emergency with an associated mortality rate of up to 10 per cent. It may be precipitated by stress and infection. Features include weight loss, oligomenorrhoea, hypercalcaemia (caused by high bone turnover) and diarrhoea. Patients are investigated with TSH and T_4 (thyroxine) levels. Treatment is supportive with cooling and rehydration. β Blockers provide symptomatic relief. Carbimazole and potassium iodide may be indicated.
- Malignant hyperpyrexia (not listed in the mnemonic) is a rare autosomal dominant disorder in which hyperpyrexia is precipitated by anaesthetic agents (e.g. halothane).

Hyperuricaemia

Really **H**igh **L**evels **P**romote **G**out

   Renal failure (chronic, lead poisoning, diuretics)

   Haemolysis

   Lesch–Nyhan syndrome

   Purine biosynthesis/**P**olycythaemia rubra vera (PRV)

   G6PD deficiency (von Gierke's disease)

Topic facts

The causes of hyperuricaemia are summarized in this mnemonic.

- Hyperuricaemia is the result of a high level of uric acid production or impaired uric acid excretion.

- Failure of uric acid clearance occurs in renal failure and with the use of diuretics. Thiazide diuretics in particular impair uric acid clearance and promote gout.

- Haemolysis, glucose-6-phosphate dehydrogenase (G6PD) deficiency and PRV are examples in which there is an increased purine load resulting in hyperuricaemia.

- Lesch–Nyhan syndrome is an X-linked recessive condition resulting from a deficiency of the enzyme hypoxanthine–guanine phosphoribosyl transferase. There is an accumulation of precursors that break down to form uric acid. Patients present with gout and renal impairment as a result of uric acid crystal formation in the kidneys.

- Uric acid is a waste product of the metabolism of purines. The purines (adenosine and guanine) and pyrimidines (thymine and cytosine) are key constituents of DNA. Hence in states of rapid cell turnover, there is a large purine load.

- G6PD deficiency is an X-linked deficiency of the enzyme G6PD which results in a haemolytic anaemia and subsequent purine load (see pages 3 and 213).

Hypocalcaemia
Parathyroid hormone/Vitamin D deficiency/Drugs

Parathyroid hormone
- Hypoparathyroidism
  - inherited
  - acquired
- Pseudohypoparathyroidism
- Hypomagnesaemia

Vitamin D deficiency
- Nutritional
- Inherited
- Renal failure
- Malabsorption

Drugs
- Oestrogens
- Bisphosphonates
- Doxorubicin
- Ketoconazole

Topic facts
The common causes of hypocalcaemia are summarized here in three categories.
- Parathyroid hormone (PTH) deficiency can be inherited (DiGeorge syndrome) or acquired after trauma or surgery, in which case it may be transient.
- Pseudohypoparathyroidism is an inherited G-protein abnormality leading to resistance to PTH.
- Magnesium is an important cofactor in the production of PTH. Hypocalcaemia persists despite calcium and vitamin D supplementation.
- Causes of vitamin D deficiency are listed under the category heading. Vitamin D is one of the fat-soluble vitamins (E, D, A and K) and may therefore be affected by malabsorption.

Hypokalaemia

Many **D**iuretics **G**enerate **R**eversible **H**ypokalaemia

Mineralocorticoid excess
- Exogenous
- Fludrocortisone
- Liquorice
- Renal tubular acidosis (RTA)

Diuretics

Gastrointestinal losses
- Vomiting
- Diarrhoea
- Fistula
- Ileostomy

Redistribution
- Alkalosis
- Insulin
- β Agonists

Hyperaldosteronism

Topic facts

This mnemonic lists the common causes of hypokalaemia.
- The mineralocorticoids, such as aldosterone, promote sodium retention in exchange for potassium loss.
- Liquorice inhibits an enzyme that prevents corticosteroids from activating mineralocorticoid receptors. This promotes an aldosterone-like effect.
- Alkalosis leads to an intracellular movement of K^+ in exchange for H^+. The reverse is true in acidosis.
- If acidosis and hypokalaemia are present, think RTA!
- Gastrointestinal secretions are potassium rich.

Metabolic acidosis

Bicarbonate loss
Bicarbonate production failure
Acid excess

Bicarbonate loss
- Diarrhoeal disorders
- Proximal renal tubular acidosis (RTA)
- Hyperparathyroidism

Bicarbonate production failure
- Distal RTA
- Spironolactone/amiloride
- Hyporeninaemic hypoaldosteronism
- Carbonic anhydrase inhibitors (acetazolamide or Diamox)

Acid excess
- Lactic
- Ketone
- Renal failure (uric acid)
- Ammonia
- Ingestion of acids (salicylate, methanol, ethylene glycol)

Topic facts
Metabolic acidosis is defined as a pH < 7.35 in the presence of a low serum bicarbonate. The causes are categorized here for easy recall.
- Metabolic acidosis is associated with hyperkalaemia, caused by a redistribution of electrolytes.
- Serum H^+ moves into cells down a concentration gradient and is exchanged for K^+.
- RTA is the exception with hypokalaemia. In type 2 RTA, loss of Na^+ activates the renin–angiotensin–aldosterone system and promotes Na^+ retention at the expense of K^+ loss.

Metabolic alkalosis

Acid loss/Low potassium

Acid loss
- Gastric acid loss
- Ingestion of alkali – rare

Low potassium
- Potassium deficit
- Hyperaldosteronism
- Bartter's syndrome
- Thiazide diuretics

Topic facts
Metabolic alkalosis is defined as a pH >7.45 in the presence of an elevated serum bicarbonate. Causes are divided into acid loss and low potassium.
- Metabolic alkalosis results from the direct loss of H^+ (or ingestion of alkali – rare) or hypokalaemia.
- Metabolic alkalosis is less common than metabolic acidosis.
- Respiratory compensation is poor because the result would be hypoxia.
- An overall potassium deficit in the body leads to conservation of K^+. The kidney reabsorbs K^+ in exchange for H^+ with resultant alkalosis.
- Bartter's syndrome is associated with K^+ loss (see page 211).
- Alkalosis leads to hypokalaemia as a result of redistribution of electrolytes. H^+ moves out of cells to buffer the plasma pH and, in exchange, K^+ moves into the cells. The converse effect is true of acidosis.
- Hypokalaemia leads to alkalosis *and* alkalosis leads to hypokalaemia.
- Carcinoma of the bronchus with ectopic ACTH production may present with hypokalaemic allcalosis.

Slow acetylators
SHIP
Sulphonamide
Hydralazine
Isoniazid
Procainamide

Topic facts
Drugs that may cause adverse side-effects in patients who are slow acetylators are summarized above.

- Genetic polymorphisms lead to significant differences in levels of drug exposure. As a result, individuals with certain phenotypes are predisposed to the development of adverse reactions.
- The slow acetylator phenotype is a common genetic polymorphism that affects up to 50 per cent of the population in the UK.
- Patients who are of the slow acetylator phenotype are at increased risk of developing isoniazid toxicity and drug-induced lupus.
- Isoniazid toxicity results because isoniazid clearance is impaired leading to higher than normal plasma levels. Patients may complain of peripheral neuropathy-type symptoms.
- Drug-induced lupus mimics the presentation of systemic lupus erythematosus (SLE); however, on withdrawal of the causative drug, symptoms resolve within days to months.
- The most common causative drugs of drug-induced lupus are listed in the mnemonic.
- The autoantibody profile of drug-induced lupus is similar to that of SLE, with positive anti-nuclear antibodies and anti-histone antibodies. However, anti-dsDNA is uncommon in drug-induced lupus.
- Drug-induced lupus tends to present in an older age group (>50) compared with SLE (average age about 30).

Syndrome of inappropriate ADH secretion

Pituitary **T**rauma **D**ilutes **B**lood

Pulmonary
- TB
- Infection
- Positive-pressure ventilation

Tumours
- Lung
- Thyroid
- Pancreas
- Bladder
- Lymphoma

Drugs
- ACE inhibitors
- Tricyclics
- Pherothriazines
- Omeprazole

Brain
- Trauma
- Tumour
- Infection
- Porphyria
- Raised intracranial pressure

Topic facts

Causes of syndrome of inappropriate ADH secretion (SIADH) are given above.

- ADH is released from the posterior pituitary in response to changes in plasma osmolality and volume. SIADH is the inappropriate release of ADH in a euvolaemic patient.
- Patients may complain of headaches, nausea and vomiting, and later develop an acute confusional state.
- Biochemical findings are of low serum sodium and osmolality with an inappropriately concentrated urine.

Tetany
Too much breathing or too few salts

Hyperventilation
Hypocalcaemia
Hypomagnesaemia
Hypokalaemia

Topic facts
This mnemonic lists the more common causes of tetany.
- Tetany is the periodic involuntary spasm of muscle as a result of neural hyperexcitability. It is often described by patients as muscle cramps.
- Tetany is caused by a disequilibrium of ionized serum calcium, which may be precipitated by hyperventilation, hypocalcaemia, hypomagnesaemia or hypokalaemia.
- Patients with panic attacks may complain of paraesthesiae and tetany. The hyperventilation results in a respiratory alkalosis. Alkalosis causes tetany by decreasing the amount of ionized calcium available in the serum.
- Magnesium is an important cofactor required for the release of PTH, which maintains serum calcium levels, and hence a deficiency may lead to hypocalcaemia.
- Trousseau's sign is the induction of tetany through restriction of blood flow in a limb by inflating a blood pressure cuff above systolic pressure. Rapid onset of tetany is used as a bedside measure of neural hyperexcitability.
- Chvostek's sign is a similar measure – tapping over the facial nerve anterior to the tragus of the ear induces tetany of the muscles of the eye, mouth and nose.
- Investigation is for causes of hypocalcaemia (see page 201).

Genetics

- Autosomal dominant conditions
- Autosomal recessive conditions
- Bartter's syndrome
- Trinucleotide repeat disorders
- X-linked recessive disorders

Autosomal dominant conditions
Noble **P**arents **W**on't **T**ransmit **M**ajor **H**ereditary **G**enetic **D**isorders

Neurofibromatosis: chromosomes 17 + 22
Porphyria (acute intermittent): chromosome 11
von **W**illebrand's disease: chromosome 12
Tuberous sclerosis: chromosome 16
Marfan syndrome/**M**yotonic dystrophy: chromosomes 15 + 19
Huntington's disease: chromosome 4
Gilbert's syndrome: chromosome 2
Dwarfism (achondroplasia): chromosome 4

Topic facts
This mnemonic lists the most common autosomal dominant conditions.
- Autosomal dominant conditions are inherited by 50 per cent of children from affected parents.
- Phenotypic abnormalities are common in autosomal dominant conditions, e.g. neurofibromas, dwarfism, marfanoid skeletal change, myopathic facies.
- Individuals may inherit the affected gene but not express features of the disorder as a result of non-penetrance.
- New mutations can lead to an autosomal dominant condition in a patient with normal parents, e.g. neurofibromatosis.
- Huntington's disease and myotonic dystrophy are trinucleotide repeat disorders (see trinucleotide repeat disorders on page 212).
- Acute intermittent porphyria (chromosome 11), variegate (chromosome 1) and co-proporphyria (chromosome 3) are all autosomal dominant.
- Gilbert's syndrome is a condition that affects up to 5 per cent of the population. It results in the intermittent elevation of bilirubin at times of stress or illness.
- Other common MRCP autosomal dominant conditions include Osler-Weber-Rendu syndrome, familial polyposis coli and Peutz-Jeghers syndrome (pg 188).

Autosomal recessive conditions
Most metabolic disorders

Examples
- Phenylketonuria
- Gaucher's disease
- Osteogenesis imperfecta
- β-Thalassaemia
- Cystic fibrosis
- Homocystinuria
- Spinal muscular atrophy
- Alkaptonuria
- Oculocutaneous albinism
- Fanconi's anaemia
- Congenital adrenal hyperplasia
- Galactosaemia
- Dubin–Johnson syndrome
- Ataxia telangiectasia

Topic facts
Common autosomal recessive disorders are shown above.
- Most metabolic disorders are autosomal recessive. The metal storage disorders haemochromatosis and Wilson's disease are also autosomal recessive.
- Learn the mnemonics for autosomal dominant and X-linked disorders. If the condition is metabolic and does not fit into the other mnemonics, the chances are that it is autosomal recessive.
- Autosomal recessive conditions are inherited by 25 per cent of children from carrier parents. Male and female offspring have an equal chance of being affected.
- Cystic fibrosis is the most common autosomal recessive condition in the UK.
- There is increased risk of both parents being carriers for the same recessive gene in parents who are closely blood-related.

Bartter's syndrome

Little	Bart's	Low salt
Recessive	Bartter's syndrome	low Na$^+$, K$^+$, H$^+$

Topic facts

Bartter's syndrome is an autosomal recessive inherited disease of childhood. The features of Bartter's syndrome are summarized above. It is a rare condition but common to the MRCP.

- There is impaired sodium chloride (NaCl) reabsorption in the loop of the kidneys. The loss of NaCl stimulates renin and aldosterone secretion, resulting in juxtaglomerular hyperplasia.
- A high level of NaCl in the collecting ducts stimulates both K$^+$ and H$^+$ secretion. This results in hypokalaemic metabolic alkalosis.
- Despite high levels of renin and aldosterone these patients have a normal blood pressure, which is thought to result from faster kinin and prostaglandin secretion.
- Treatments involve replacement of salts with oral supplements and prostaglandin inhibitors (e.g. indometacin) to oppose the elevated prostaglandin levels.

Trinucleotide repeat disorders

Hunt **M**ultiple **F**ragile **S**equences

   Huntington's disease

   Myotonic dystrophy

   Friedreich's ataxia/**F**ragile **X**

   Spinocerebellar ataxia

Topic facts

The trinucleotide repeat disorders are a group of inherited disorders with a common pathological process. Common examples are listed above.

- The trinucleotide repeat disorders have a varied inheritance pattern.
- The abnormality is the result of genes that contain multiple repeating units in which each unit comprises three nucleotides.
- As the disorder is passed on to the next generation the number of trinucleotide repeats increases. This leads to the phenomenon called anticipation.
- Anticipation is the increase in the severity of the condition and presentation of the disease at an earlier age in successive generations of affected individuals.
- Huntington's disease, myotonic dystrophy and spinocerebellar ataxia are all autosomal dominant.
- Friedreich's ataxia is autosomal recessive.
- Fragile X syndrome is X-linked recessive.

X-linked recessive disorders

Blame **D**iseased **G**irls

  Bleeding disorders: haemophilia A + B

  Duchenne muscular dystrophy

  G6PD deficiency

Topic facts

Common X-linked disorders are summarized in this topic.

- X-linked recessive disorders result from a recessive mutation on the X chromosome.
- X-linked recessive disorders typically affect males only.
- Males inherit only one copy of the X gene (from their mother – blame diseased girls). So if a mutation is present it will be expressed.
- Heterozygous females are carriers of the gene.
- An affected man cannot pass disease to his sons (as sons of a man inherit his Y chromosome).
- All daughters of an affected man are carriers (as daughters of a man inherit his X chromosome).
- A carrier female passes the affected gene to 50 per cent of her sons and 50 per cent of her daughters. Hence 50 per cent of her daughters will be carriers and 50 per cent of her sons will be affected.
- Females can be affected in the following circumstances:
  - patient with Turner syndrome (XO) inherits an affected X chromosome
  - atypical lyonization (the patient typically has a milder form of the disease).

General

- Bony metastasis
- Clubbing
- Dermatomes, myotomes and reflexes
- Dupuytren's contracture
- Genital ulcers

Bony metastasis

Spine **P**articularly **R**iddled
  Spine
  Pelvis
  Ribs
  Skull
  Proximal long bones

Renal **T**umours **P**enetrate **B**one
  Renal
  Thyroid
  Prostate
  Breast/**B**ronchial

Topic facts

The sites involved by bony metastasis, with the most common listed first, are given in the first mnemonic. The second lists the cancers that commonly metastasize to bone.

- Breast and prostate cancer are the most common causes of bony metastasis, accounting for up to two-thirds of all cases.
- Complications of bony metastasis:
  - pathological fracture
  - hypercalcaemia
  - bone pain
  - disfigurement.
- Management of bone pain can be difficult and the following principles should be followed:
  - regular preventive medication is more effective than as-required medication
  - NSAIDs, bisphosphonates and radiotherapy are of particular benefit in bony metastasis.

General

Clubbing
Cardiac/Respiratory/Abdominal

Cardiac
ACE
Atrial myxoma
Cyanotic congenital heart disease
Endocarditis

Respiratory
Scarring Causes Clubbing
Suppurative
- Bronchiectasis
- Empyema
- Lung abscess

Cancers
- Mesothelioma
- Bronchial neoplasm

Cryptogenic fibrosing alveolitis (and other causes of lung fibrosis)

Abdominal
4 Cs
Cirrhosis
Crohn's disease
Coeliac disease
Chronic disease

Topic facts
The causes of clubbing, categorized by system, are shown above.
- Conditions that mimic the appearance of clubbing:
  - thyroid acropachy
  - terminal resorption of the phalanges (as a result of chronic hyperparathyroidism, look for a neck scar of parathyroidectomy).

Dermatomes, myotomes and reflexes

- Knowledge of dermatomes, myotomes and reflex roots is essential for tackling MRCP clinical problems. Unfortunately these facts have to be learnt by rote. The next few pages include some memory aids to help rapid recall of these facts.

(Dermatomes of the legs and arms)

You stand on S1
You sit on S3
The first three lumbars go down to the knee
L4 on the inside
L5 on the out
S3 on the bits you shake about!

    S1 supplies the sole of the feet
    S3 supplies the bottom
    L1 supplies top of the leg, L2 the thigh and L3 the knee
    L4 supplies the medial aspect of the shin
    L5 supplies the lateral aspect
    S3 supplies the perineum

Topic facts

The dermatomal distribution of the legs is summarized in this memory aid.

- Unfortunately I have no mnemonic for the upper arms. The dermatomal distribution is outlined below for your information.
- The shoulder starts at C4, then C5 supplies the lateral aspect of the proximal arm, C6 the lateral part of the forearm, thumb and first finger, C7 the middle finger, and C8 the fourth and fifth digits. T1 supplies the medial aspect of the forearm and T2 the medial aspect of the proximal arm.
- The first cervical dermatome is C2 (occiput); C3 supplies the neck.

Dermatomes, myotomes and reflexes (continued)

(Muscular innervation of the arms)

General

Chicken, Pull, Push, Grab, Spread
Lift and Pinch

Chicken: C4 (abduction of arms)

Pull: C5, 6 (biceps, flexion)

Push: C7 (triceps extension)

Grab: C8 (finger flexion)

Spread: T1, ulnar (finger abduction)

Lift and Pinch: median nerve (thumb abduction and opposition)

(Chicken refers to the position where the arms are held parallel to the shoulders with elbows bent downwards towards the hips. Press downwards on the upper arm to test abduction. Movement of the elbows anteriorly and posteriorly in this position makes you flap like a chicken!)

Topic facts

The myotomal distribution in the upper limbs is summarized here.

- The small muscles of the hand (palmar and dorsal interossei) are supplied by the ulnar nerve. The action of the muscles is recalled using the common mnemonics PAD and DAB. Palmar muscles **AD**-duct (PAD) the **D**orsal muscles **AB**-duct (DAB).

Dermatomes, myotomes and reflexes (continued)

(Muscular innervation of the legs)

Twelve, twelve, thirty-four,
one, forty-five
Hip (flexion): L**1, 2**
Knee (flexion): S**1, 2**
Knee (extension): L**3, 4**
Ankle (plantarflexion): S**1**
Ankle (dorsiflexion): L**4, 5**

General

Topic facts
It is best to learn the myotomes off by heart and use a fixed routine to examine them. This allows for a rapid and slick assessment. To remember which nerves are 'L' and which are 'S' the order is alphabetical (i.e. starts with L) and then alternates.
- L4, 5 lesions cause foot drop – this is the common peroneal nerve.
- Foot drop can be a result of trauma as the nerve winds around the head of the fibula – classically caused by bumper damage from a car. Other causes are the same as for other mononeuropathies.

Dermatomes, myotomes and reflexes (continued)

Reflexes

Ankle, Knee and SB, T
Ankle: S1, 2
Knee: L3, 4
Supinator: C5, 6
Biceps: C5, 6
Triceps: C7

Topic facts
The reflexes are relatively easy to recall because there is a clear numerical pattern and the part of the spine (i.e. lumbar/thoracic/cervical) changes on each reflex until you reach the cervical level.
- If reflexes are absent, reinforcement techniques should be used to try to elicit a response. Examples include asking the patient to grasp the hands together and pull apart just before stimulating the reflex. Another method is to ask the patient to grit the teeth.
- When assessing spinal cord damage you should assess the reflex, motor and sensory level of involvement (see pages 72 and 79).

Dupuytren's contracture
SHAME

Smoking

HIV/AIDS

Alcohol and liver disease

Manual labour

Endocrine (diabetes)/**E**pileptic drugs (phenytoin)

Topic facts
Dupuytren's contracture is disease resulting in fixed flexion contractures of the fingers. This mnemonic lists the associated causes.

- The disease process is thought to result from oxidization and fibrosis of the palmar fascia.
- The ring finger is the most commonly affected digit.
- Dupuytren's contracture is most common in white individuals.
- Men are more commonly affected than women.
- Contractures usually present after the age of 50.
- Management includes surgical release for those with a contracture leading to disability. No medical management has been shown to be effective.
- Dupuytren's contracture is a member of a group of diseases called the fibromatoses which include Peyronie's disease (penile fibromatosis – bent penile shaft).

General

Genital ulcers
Contagious Ladies Have Smelly Genitals
Don't Bonk Them

Infectious
Chancroid
Lymphogranuloma venereum
Herpes simplex/HIV-specific ulcers
Syphilis
Granuloma inguinale

Non-infectious
Drugs
Behçet's syndrome
Trauma

Topic facts
This topic divides the causes of genital ulcers into infectious and
non-infectious.
- Chanchroid (*Haemophilus ducreyi*) is a sexually transmitted infection (STI)
  characterized by the presence of painful ulcers and inguinal
  lymphadenopathy. Investigation is with Gram stain and culture (although
  polymerase chain reaction [PCR] can be used). Treatment is with
  antibiotics after determination of sensitivity.
- Lymphogranuloma (venereum) (LGV) is an STI common in tropical
  climates (Africa, India, South America). Inguinal lymphadenopathy may
  develop. Test for serology.
- HIV-specific ulcers can occur during the acute infection phase or later in
  the disease course.
- Syphilis (*Treponema pallidum*) presents with a painless ulcer (chancre)
  that is infectious. Syphilis is largely penicillin sensitive (see page 179).
- Granuloma inguinale is an STI of tropical origin. Treat with tetracycline.

Exam technique

Exam technique – Part 1

Key principles for passing Part 1
- Multiple choice questions (MCQs) are the best form of revision for the Part 1 (if you can answer the MCQs you can pass Part 1!).
- Use this book as a reference tool as you go through your practice questions, to provide you with memory aids, key facts and lists on the topic that you are reading.
- Avoid reading through a textbook of medicine. This takes a long time and is not a good way of retaining information. If you want to read a text, get a core textbook aimed directly at the MRCP Part 1 syllabus. See the recommended resources below.
- Score your practice MCQs as you go along and identify topics in which you score poorly. Concentrate on the major topics and those in which you score poorly in order to maximize your learning curve. (We all like answering questions on topics that we are good at, but this does not maximize improvement.)
- MRCP Part 1 largely relies on getting through a large number of questions; however, discussion of difficult topics with colleagues can improve understanding and aid motivation.
- The best way of passing the MRCP is first time, because having to put all the time, money and effort in on second and subsequent attempts is stressful. Avoid 'practice' attempts, plan how you want to revise and allow the time necessary.

Why use exam revision courses?
- Utilizing course study leave maximizes your time for revision.
- Courses are extremely focused and help you to cover a large amount of revision in a concentrated space of time.
- Not only will a course provide information in your favoured learning style but in a variety of other learning styles that will augment your learning process (lectures, oral discussion, group question solving, practice papers, homework questions, slides).

- Courses enable you to compare your progress with that of your colleagues through homework and practice papers.
- Practice papers under exam conditions help you to gauge the amount of time that you have on each question.

Basic MCQ technique

- Read the instructions sent in the post and ensure that you bring the required documentation (otherwise you will have an expensive day trip for nothing).
- Read the instructions on the paper carefully, ensuring that you fill in your details clearly on all documents.
- Quickly confirm how many questions there are in the paper so that you can pace yourself to finish on time.
- Read the questions in full before answering. Some candidates find it useful to cover the answers and think of the correct answer before they can be distracted by the others.
- Pay careful attention to phrases such as *commonly*, *rarely* or *sometimes*. Changing a single word can change the answer to the question.
- Statements such as *always* and *never* are usually false (but not 'always')!

Recommended resources for Part 1

- Online questions: www.onexamination.com
- MRCP Part 1-focused text: Philip A Kalra. *Essential Revision Notes for MRCP*, 2nd edn. Knutsford, Cheshire: PasTest, 2004.
- Exam course: *PasTest MRCP Part 1 Course*
- MCQ revision questions:
  - Geraint Rees. *MRCP 1: 300 Best of Five Questions and Answers* Knutsford: PasTest, 2003.
  - Helen Fellows et al. *Best of Five Questions for MRCP Part 1* (MRCP Study Guides). Knutsford: PasTest, 2003.

Exam technique – Part 2

Key principles for passing Part 2

The key principles for passing Part 2 are the same as for Part 1.
- Practise as many questions as possible.
- Read the recommended text.
- Use this book as a reference to provide you with memory aids, key facts and lists on the topics that appear in the MCQs.
- Score your MCQs and concentrate on major topics and poor scoring areas.
- Plan time for revision and courses.
- Take a course to maximize your learning time and progress.

Recommended resources for Part 2
- Online questions: www.onexamination.com
- MRCP Part 2-focused text: Sanjay Sharma and Rashmi Kaushal. *Rapid Review of Clinical Medicine for MRCP Part 2*. Oxford: Blackwell, 2006.
- Exam course: Sharma, Part 2 course (see above)
- MCQ revision questions: N. Bajaj. *Self Assessment for the MRCP Part 2 Written Paper*, Vols 1–3. Oxford: Blackwell Science Ltd, 2001.

Exam technique – PACES

Key principles for passing PACES

- Start by reading the recommended text and learning the examination routines. Correct and adapt your examination technique. Learn it by heart and practise it regularly (it is easiest to do this with partners, but large teddy bears will suffice if partners are unavailable).
- Once the examination routines are automatic and rapid, you should get into the habit of completing the correct technique on every patient whom you examine. If you have become competent it should not take much longer to rattle off a complete system examination rather than your previous examination routine. If time is too short for this, choose the most relevant examination routine and complete it in full.
- Use this book as a reference aid as you see cases, to provide you with memory aids and key facts on the examination, signs, differential diagnosis and common exam questions.
- Use the reference text (see recommended resources for PACES) as a checklist, and try to see all the cases listed within it. Outpatient clinics are often a good resource for locating the necessary clinical signs. Ask on-call doctors to record patients with interesting signs on the medical assessment ward so that you can review them on the wards.
- Find a friendly registrar who has just passed the MRCP, to watch you examine and quiz you after.
- Attend a PACES course early to assess the required standard and compare your level of competence. Based on this you can assess your deficiencies and plan your learning.
- Familiarity with your exam routines, clothes and environment will relax you and improve your confidence and performance. As the exam approaches practise your routines on patients while dressed in your exam clothes (a smart suit/dress). Equipment will be in unfamiliar pockets, which can upset your exam routine and train of thought.
- If possible visit the exam location so you are aware of the journey time, parking and location of the exam room. This will help you to be more comfortable on your second visit!
- Obtain the essential equipment and carry it with you on the wards.

- Essential equipment:
  - tendon hammer
  - stethoscope
  - ophthalmoscope
  - cotton wool
  - orange pin
  - neurological pinprick tool
  - coins.

In the exam

- Always introduce yourself and shake the patient's hand at the start of the examination, and thank the patient at the end of the physical examination before you take questions from the examiner.
- Avoid annoying patients at all costs. If they fail to cooperate patients can make their signs difficult to find. On the other hand, if they like you they may offer the area in which the sign is to be found. The patients who come to PACES are doing so to help you out – they don't get paid much and we are indebted to them.
- Presentation is extremely important. The ideal candidate is smartly dressed, confident (but not cocky), knowledgeable and polite.
- When answering questions face the examiner (after having thanked the patient) and stand with your hands behind your back and stethoscope in your hands (not round your neck). Look at the examiner who is talking to you and avoid looking back at the patient (you should have confirmed your findings before the discussion starts).
- While examining, your mind should be considering the possible diagnosis, not the next step in the routine.
- As you examine each finding make a conscious decision on whether the sign is present or absent. You should not have to repeat a part of the examination. This gives the appearance of poor examination skills and lack of practice and confidence.
- Be ready to discuss the clinical findings as soon as you have finished your physical examination. Once you have elicited the clinical finding, use the time going through the motions of completing the examination to prepare for the questions.
- Consider examining the lungs from the back before you examine the front. This is where the largest surface area of lung can be examined and where most of the clinical findings are present in respiratory cases. If you run out of time and you have examined only the front you may be stuck!

A smooth way of doing this is to assess the lymph nodes in the neck from behind and then move on to examine the back of the chest while they are in the forward position.
- If you get sweaty palms when you are nervous, try using some antiperspirant on them!
- When you have finished one station do not waste time. Put it out of your mind and start preparing for the next by recalling the 10 most common cases. In this way your mind will be in gear to face its next challenge.
- If cases are rare you may pass even if you don't get the diagnosis as long as you discuss your clinical findings in a logical fashion.
- When asked for investigations consider that all investigations are available to you, but start with simple ones and then move up the chain.

Recommended resources for Part 2
- MRCP PACES-focused text:
  - R. E. J. Ryder, M. A. Mir and E. A. Freeman. *An Aid to the MRCP PACES*. Vol. 1, *Stations 1, 3 and 5*, 3rd edn. Oxford: Blackwell, 2003.
  - R. E. J. Ryder, M. A. Mir and E. A. Freeman. *An Aid to the MRCP PACES*. Vol. 2, *Stations 1, 3 and 5*, 3rd edn. Oxford: Blackwell, 2003.
- Exam course:
  - PasTest PACES 5-day course
  - PACES ahead weekend course
- Outpatient clinics
- Medical assessment unit
- Wards
- Specialist registrars.

After you have sat an attempt at PACES
- Please visit www.ryder.MRCP.org.uk and fill in the on-line survey. This will be used for future editions of An Aid to the MRCP PACES and help future candidates, just as the candidates in past surveys have helped you.

Appendix

Summary of abbreviations

5-FU	5-fluorouracil (chemotherapy agent)
α_1AT	α_1-antitrypsin deficiency
ABG	arterial blood gas
ACE	angiotensin-converting enzyme
ACTH	adrenocorticotrophic hormone
ADH	antidiuretic hormone
AF	atrial fibrillation
AIDS	acquired immune deficiency syndrome
AIP	acute intermittent porphyria
ALA	aminolaevulinic acid
ALL	acute lymphoblastic leukaemia
ANA	anti-nuclear antibody
AML	acute myeloid leukaemia
ANCA	anti-neutrophil cytoplasmic antibody
APCKD	adult polycystic kidney disease
APPT	activated partial thromboplastin time
ASD	atrial septal defect
ASOT	anti-streptolysin O titre
ATN	acute tubular necrosis
AV	atrioventricular or arteriovenous
BCG	bacille Calmette–Guérin
BHL	bilateral hilar lymphadenopathy
BSE	bovine spongiform encephalopathy
BT	bleeding time
CAH	congenital adrenal hyperplasia or chronic active hepatitis
cAMP	adenosine cyclic 3′:5′-monophosphate
CDI	cranial diabetes insipidus
CJD	Creutzfeldt–Jakob disease
CLL	chronic lymphatic leukaemia
CML	chronic myeloid leukaemia
CMV	cytomegalovirus

CNS	central nervous system
COPD	chronic obstructive pulmonary disease
COX-1	cyclo-oxygenase 1
CREST	calcinosis, Raynaud's phenomenon, oesophagitis, sclerosis, telangiectasia
CRP	C-reactive protein
CT	computed tomography
CTS	carpal tunnel syndrome
CVA	cerebrovascular accident
DHEA	dihydroepiandosterone (steroid precursor)
DIC	disseminated intravascular coagulation
DIP	distal interphalangeal
DMARD	disease-modifying anti-rheumatoid drug
DVLA	Driver and Vehicle Licensing Agency
EBV	Epstein–Barr virus
ECG	electrocardiogram
EN	erythema nodosum
ERCP	endoscopic retrograde cholangiopancreatography
ESR	erythrocyte sedimentation rate
FBC	full blood count
FSH	follicle-stimulating hormone
FTA-Abs	fluorescent treponemal antibody absorption test
G6PD	glucose-6-phosphate dehydrogenase
GBS	Guillain–Barré syndrome
GI	gastrointestinal
GTN	glyceryl trinitrate
HAART	highly active antiretroviral therapy
HDL	high-density lipoprotein
HIT	heparin-induced thrombocytopenia
HIV	human immunodeficiency virus
HLA	human leukocyte antigen (found on chromosome 6)
HSP	Henoch–Schönlein purpura
HUS	haemolytic uraemic syndrome
IBD	inflammatory bowel disease
ICP	intracranial pressure
IDL	intermediate-density lipoprotein
Ig	immunoglobulin
INR	international normalized ratio
ITP	idiopathic thrombocytopenic purpura

JVP	jugular venous pressure
LDL	low-density lipoprotein
LH	luteinizing hormone
LMN	lower motor neuron
LV	left ventricle
LVF	left ventricular failure
MACGN	mesangiocapillary glomerulonephritis
MCP	metacarpophalangeal
MCV	mean corpuscular volume
MDMA	3,4-methylene dioxymetamphetamine
MEN	multiple endocrine neoplasia
MHA	microangiopathic haemolytic anaemia
MI	myocardial infarction
MMR	measles, mumps, rubella (triple vaccine)
MND	motor neuron disease
MPA	microscopic polyangitis
MRI	magnetic resonance imaging
MS	multiple sclerosis
NAP	neutrophil alkaline phosphatase
NDI	nephrogenic diabetes insipidus
NRTI	nucleoside reverse transcriptase inhibitor
NSAID	non-steroidal anti-inflammatory drug
PAN	polyarteritis nodosa
PBC	primary biliary cirrhosis
PCOS	polycystic ovary syndrome
PCP	*Pneumocystis carinii* pneumonia
PCR	polymerase chain reaction
PCV	packed cell volume
PE	pulmonary embolism
PGAD	polyglandular autoimmune disease
pH	measure of acidity
PI	protease inhibitor
PMR	polymyalgia rheumatica
PNH	paroxysmal nocturnal haemoglobinuria
PPH	primary pulmonary hypertension
PPI	proton pump inhibitor
PRV	polycythaemia rubra vera
PSC	primary sclerosing cholangitis
PTH	parathyroid hormone

Appendix

PTHrp	PTH-related peptide
PUVA	psoralen + ultraviolet (light) A
QRS	QRS complex on an ECG (ventricular contraction)
RAPD	relative afferent pupillary defect
RBC	red blood cell
RNP	ribonucleoprotein
RTA	renal tubular acidosis
RV	right ventricle
RVH	right ventricular hypertrophy
SAAG	serum ascites albumin gradient
SAH	subarachnoid haemorrhage
SBE	subacute bacterial endocarditis
SBP	spontaneous bacterial peritonitis
SDH	subdural haemorrhage
SIADH	syndrome of inappropriate ADH secretion
SLE	systemic lupus erythematosus
SMA	smooth muscle antibody
SOL	space-occupying lesion
T_4	thyroxine
TB	tuberculosis
TD	tardive dyskinesia
TIA	transient ischaemic attack
TNF	tumour necrosis factor
TRH	thyroid hormone-releasing hormone
TSE	transmissible spongiform encephalopathy
TSH	thyroid-stimulating hormone
TT	thrombin time
TTP	thrombotic thrombocytopenic purpura
UC	ulcerative colitis
UMN	upper motor neuron
VLDL	very-low-density lipoprotein
VDRL	Venereal Disease Research Laboratory
VSD	ventricular septal defect
VT	ventricular tachycardia
WBC	white blood cell
WCC	white cell count
WPW	Wolff–Parkinson–White

Appendix

Index

Index

Index